THE LIVING OF THESE DAYS

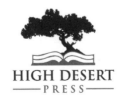

HIGH DESERT
—— P R E S S ——

Order
From: **Cozy Nook**
11655 E Albert Rd
Rich Hill, MO 64779

High Desert Press
26 Road 5577
Farmington, NM 87401
highdesertpress@gmail.com

ISBN: 978-1-7923-5236-2

Printed in the United States of America

First Printing: November 2020

God of Grace and God of Glory

God of grace and God of glory,
On Thy people pour Thy pow'r;
Crown Thine ancient church's story
Bring her bud to glorious flow'r.
Grant us wisdom, Grant us courage,
For the facing of this hour,
For the facing of this hour.

Lo! the hosts of evil round us
Scorn Thy Christ, assail His ways!
From the fears that long have bound us,
Free our hearts to faith and praise.
Grant us wisdom, Grant us courage,
For the living of these days,
For the living of these days.

Cure Thy children's warring madness;
Bend our pride to Thy control;
Shame our wanton, selfish gladness,
Rich in things and poor in soul.
Grant us wisdom, Grant us courage,
Lest we miss Thy kingdom's goal,
Lest we miss Thy kingdom's goal.

Table of Contents

Introduction

I DON'T REMEMBER ever hearing or seeing the word *pandemic* before COVID-19. It wasn't a new word, just one I didn't know or need until 2020.

When reports of a novel coronavirus began to appear in the newspaper around the beginning of the year, I didn't pay much attention to them for a few months. But when it began affecting my life, including my job as a caregiver at an assisted living home, I started paying attention.

After doing some research, I learned that a cluster of unusual pneumonia cases had been discovered near Wuhan, China, in December 2019. The virus that caused the infections was named SARS-CoV-2 (severe acute respiratory syndrome coronavirus 2) and the illness that it caused received an official name—COVID-19, which stands for *coronavirus disease 2019*.

In this book, the terms *coronavirus*, *COVID*, and *COVID-19* all mean the same thing. Not all coronaviruses are COVID-19, but when it is mentioned in these stories, it is referring to the specific coronavirus that caused COVID-19.

In the travel-easy world of today, it didn't take long until the virus was carried to other countries. On January 30, 2020, the World Health Organization (WHO) declared the outbreak a public health emergency of international concern. On March 11, WHO declared it a pandemic.

In the days and weeks following March 11, nonessential businesses were forced to close, and crowd size limits grew smaller and smaller, all the way down to five in some areas. Stay-at-home orders were issued in an attempt to slow the spread of the virus. Everyone who had to be out in public was expected to practice social distancing by staying at least six feet away from anyone else. Because affected people spread the virus by droplets, masks became necessary accessories.

In the middle of May, I received a story from Sheila Petre called "Aunt Jo's Mask Factory." After reading about Aunt Jo and her unusual business, I thought about the many other unusual situations that COVID-19 brought into our lives. Could I gather stories and compile a book, thereby preserving the history of the COVID-19 pandemic and all the changes it brought to the world in 2020?

The COVID-19 health crisis was unprecedented in modern times, but in 1918, the Spanish flu swept over the world. Since the beginning of the COVID-19 pandemic, I have often wondered what life was like during the Spanish flu pandemic, especially for those of Anabaptist faith.

After receiving encouragement, advice, and suggestions from several experienced writer and publisher friends, I collected pandemic stories from Anabaptists in numerous states and multiple countries.

I hope this book will be preserved for future generations, so if they face a pandemic of COVID-19 proportions, they can learn how things were done in 2020.

—Erica Sauder

The Preacher's COVID Lessons

Rodney Witmer

My intent in sharing the following piece is not to insist on a certain view of the COVID-19 scenario, nor is it to imply that other preachers' sentiments would mirror my own. Rather, my goal is simply to share my experience.

The COVID-19 dilemma is still very much impacting the local scene. How or if it will end, only God knows. It has, however, been a valuable experience for me and for the churches. From the standpoint of sickness and loss of life, the pandemic is a sad story. But from the standpoint of the reality check it gave us all, from the aspect of the way it brought us face to face with "if the Lord will, we shall live, and do this or that," it has been invaluable.

As I write, I am sipping this pineapple-flavored beverage. It's good the container notifies me of the pineapple thing, because to my mouth, the liquid is flat and flavorless. Compliments of a personal stint with COVID-19 ten weeks ago, I still live in a tasteless, odorless world. It would be so nice to have church with everyone again—and to taste and smell things.

IT WAS WHILE our church at Farmington was grappling with the early stages of Sasha Krause's disappearance, in January 2020, that I first began to read about this coronavirus sweeping through Wuhan, China. I saw pictures of people in masks. I read about empty subways and streets, and wondered what a locked-down city was really like. It never occurred to me that such a scene would sweep like a tidal wave around the globe and into our own little high-elevation corner of it. But it did. I have never seen something go from a localized problem to a global emergency so rapidly.

I remember listening to adults pray when I was a child. They would thank the Lord for plenty of food, or religious freedom, or health, and then this curious phrase would follow: "Help us not to take this for granted." I had no idea what that meant, but could mimic the lingo long before I comprehended it.

I comprehend it better now, and I've thought about that phrase and concept a lot in the past year. My wife's cancer, Sasha's disappearance and murder, and the whole COVID scene have, I suppose, inspired most of these reflections. I realize that subconsciously, I've taken a lot for granted over the years. But life looks much more uncertain today than ever before, more tenuous, more fragile, more fleeting, and…more precious.

Our American culture, including our American conservative Mennonite culture, has existed and functioned almost unimpeded for so long that we foolishly begin to "take it for granted." In fact, we begin to feel we are entitled to it.

For the past twenty-four years, I have been a preacher in the church at Farmington, New Mexico. God has used and still is using this calling to shape, perfect, and even chastise me—all things I stand in need of.

Something happens, however, when you labor in that calling for a long time, when you put your heart into that calling, and when you seek to relate to that calling in a God-honoring way. This calling is a work among people. God loves these people. These people love God. They seek to honor and serve Him. You come to love these people, be protective of them, and be sensitive to things that seem to threaten them.

COVID-19 seemed to threaten us. It wasn't our health that felt threatened, though we are as vulnerable as anyone. But suddenly, right during the trauma of Sasha's murder, we could no longer gather and encourage one another. Right when I was trying to lead, comfort, and defend, it felt as if I couldn't.

> Lesson 1: We'll be fine because God is not boxed
> in, and His Word is not bound. I am not indis-
> pensable to our success; God is.

So, one Sunday we had gathered and packed the building as usual. The next Sunday, the building was all but empty, and I preached to a microphone while the audience listened at home.

I learned how much the audience is part of the whole preaching experience, how much faces contribute to the preacher's inspiration and delivery. The preaching of the Word is for the benefit of the people. When the people are not there, something feels awkward. Stage fright is the fear of facing an audience. I don't know what you call the feeling that goes with facing an empty auditorium.

Of course, the lack of a visible audience was only one of the factors affecting me. I prepared differently because the truth had to be conveyed entirely verbally. Facial expressions would not be seen. Gestures that come naturally only stirred the air near the pulpit and made me feel foolish when I caught myself. I wondered how the people were doing and if they were listening. When I was finished preaching, the air seemed to hang thick and unresolved. No discussion afterward. No sense of effect.

> Lesson 2: It's God's Word, not mine. It does not
> return to Him void. It accomplishes things.

We solved a bit of the awkwardness of preaching to emptiness by inviting just a handful of people to sit on the pews every Sunday. We also conducted a few drive-in services and we ministers preached from an elevated bank on the lawn. In spite of seeing more windshields than faces, it was inspirational to have the people present.

As I preached at one of those drive-in services, I had the distinct and nostalgic feeling of playing church. It was not because the service was festive or light-hearted, but because it was outside and only about five hundred feet from where I had played church as a boy and preached my first sermons. It's amazing what life can put back together.

We had an outdoor baptism for two young men and an outdoor reception for one of our couples who had been forced to have a small home wedding in Kentucky.

As I write, our governor has allowed us to resume services, beginning with 25 percent capacity and now raised to 40 percent. To give our people opportunity to go to a service every Sunday, we have conducted three or four services each Sunday for several months now. We are deeply grateful for the fellowship this has afforded us.

On a more personal note, I've had to deal with a bit of guilt. Because I care, I tend to take personally things that are beyond my control. It's interesting how that I can know the following things are beyond my control, and yet still feel guilty about them:

- Canceling church
- Organizing other methods for having church
- The inability to be scheduled with instruction classes

- The feeling I should be doing something differently but not knowing what
- Knowing I am not reaching around pastorally
- A defeat or struggle someone has experienced
- A general sense of not taking care of the flock as I should
- The altering of some forms and practices

These things are real to me, and they are probably more acute simply because they came right on the heels of the Sasha Krause tragedy. That alone had many of us feeling helplessly responsible.

But I am finding my way through all of this because God is good, and our brotherhood is solid, and my fellow ministry are God's gift to me. It has also steadied me to know that faithful churches everywhere had to deal with this pandemic.

Lesson 3: I will be held accountable only for those things within my control and power to choose. My influence and teaching must be sound, but I am not accountable for others' choices or for distresses caused by Satan and allowed by God.

Actually, I am grateful for the forced focus we've been given on what really matters. I love our faith and practice and forms of worship. But if we panic because our exact method, preferred form, or schedule is altered by circumstances beyond our control, we are probably spoiled, naive, presumptuous, and arrogant, while at the same time missing the core of what makes the church the body of Christ.

The slowed pace has been good for me, as well as finding other ways of doing what needs to be done. Saints in all times have been affected by circumstances beyond their control. Saints can prosper in any distress because of the God they serve. A kingdom not of this world can prosper in spite of this world.

> Lesson 4: God allowed the scene at hand. It must refocus us on core issues. It must shatter the false securities we have. As time goes on, there will be more interruptions in our lives, not fewer. But no man or trouble can rob us of the provisions for faithfulness.

As we long and pray for normalcy, I hope we do not miss learning any divinely intended lesson. In October 1989, the World Series baseball games were going on in the city of San Francisco when suddenly the city was shaken by a powerful earthquake. The games abruptly ended. Bridges collapsed. Buildings crumbled. Cars were crushed. People died. I remember looking at a cartoon a few days after the quake. The cartoon depicted a baseball stadium. Giant cracks had opened in the field, and the baseball players were crawling out of the cracks, adjusting their caps and yelling, "Play ball!" The implication was that we *must* get back to the all-important business at hand. We *must* return to normal. I remember shuddering at the spirit that cartoon depicted. What if God would like to alter our normal? Are we teachable and moldable?

> Lesson 5: Our responses to these events reveal whether our values, securities, and enterprises are properly premised. Can I accept a divine realignment of my world?

What am I taking for granted? Do I feel entitled to life as I have always known it? Or do I agree with James 4:14, 15: "For what is your life? It is even a vapour, that appeareth for a little time, and then vanisheth away. For that ye ought to say, If the Lord will, we shall live, and do this, or that"?

A Promise Only He Can Keep

Stephanie J. Leinbach

I SHIFTED IN my chair, wishing it were more comfortable. I was too tired to read, so I sipped vending-machine coffee and eavesdropped on nearby conversations.

The TV on the wall flashed from commercial to news. The news anchors began talking about coronavirus again. Apparently, chronic smokers were more vulnerable to this new virus from China. I wondered if the lady with the smoker's voice across the waiting room would care.

Every TV I had encountered in the last three days mentioned the virus, but I was only idly interested. Of far greater concern to me—my daughter, who was currently in the OR.

When Dr. Abel, Tarica's neurosurgeon, appeared in his blue scrubs sometime later, he motioned me from the surgical waiting area into a small consultation room. It was nearly filled by a large desk whose broad surface contained only a computer and a box of tissues. He took the empty chair in front of the computer. I slid into a chair on the opposite side of the desk and leaned my elbows on it. It was only Wednesday, but it had been a long week.

Despite his own long day, Dr. Abel looked composed, as always. "The procedure is done. Tarica is doing well. Once she wakes up, you'll be able to see her. She will be monitored in the epilepsy unit for twenty-four hours before she's discharged."

"So, we go home tomorrow night?"

"If all goes well."

Even outside the operating room, Dr. Abel was still a neuro-surgeon. Cautious. Careful. Slow to promise anything, perhaps because he knew how badly and abruptly things can go wrong. I knew, too, better than I used to. It was my job as a parent, however, to get as many answers as possible out of his reticence.

"Do you have an approximate date when surgery might happen?" I held Dr. Abel's gaze, hoping he could hear how much his answer would matter. I needed something tangible to hang onto. Not promises—epilepsy doesn't allow us the luxury of promises—but *something*. "Her seizures intensify every few months—June, September, January were all bad. January was a seizure every hour or so for most of the month. It was—" I looked away from him to stare at the tissue box until the lump dissolved in my throat. "—hard." I met his eyes again. "It's March now and she could soon have another bad month. I don't want you to think we're fine with going home to wait six weeks for surgery. I don't know if we can do another January."

Two days ago, my ten-year-old daughter had been admitted to Children's Hospital of Pittsburgh so Dr. Abel could surgically insert electrodes into her brain to locate the source of her seizures. She was taken off all medications and allowed to seize. Some of the seizures were so long and violent her left side was partially paralyzed afterward and her whole body ached.

But all those seizures had given Dr. Abel the information he needed—in two days, instead of the seven we had been told to expect. He had just removed the electrodes, and everyone considered the procedure a success.

We had agreed to move ahead with surgery that would, we hoped, remove the seizure source from her brain, despite the risks. No one knew if she would be able to use her left arm and leg post-surgery, since the seizures were originating from the area of her brain that controlled muscle movement on her left side. A heartrending risk, but Tarica was committed to taking it. With that decision made, we now wanted it over and done, the sooner the better.

Setting a date for the surgery, known as laser ablation, wasn't merely a matter of an open operating room. Special equipment needed to be flown in, and certain people needed to be present for the surgery, which could take up to seven hours.

Dr. Abel heard me but promised nothing. After all, he wasn't in charge of scheduling surgeries, only performing them. When we parted, I had nothing but the assurance that he understood how badly we needed relief.

We had a blessedly quiet night in Room EP06 and rose with a plan for the day. Linford was coming late afternoon to take us home. As eager as Tarica was to see her daddy, I knew I had to keep her busy and distracted lest she drive me to distraction.

First, breakfast. I ordered Tarica's and ran down to the cafeteria to grab mine. When I returned, Tarica had an announcement. "Dr. Abel was here. He showed me pictures of his two dogs. They are really big and came from a farm, and he doesn't know what kind they are. He said they are the biggest mistake he ever made. And he has a one-year-old baby girl."

I laid aside my frustration at missing him and laughed instead. This, this was why I liked Dr. Abel. I spent every minute of my time with him trying to extract information, and my daughter learned more than I did without trying. He *saw* her. She wasn't merely a number or a means to justify his doubtless astronomical salary. He dealt with the parents, but he was there for the children. However, he had not come to her room to discuss his misadventures in dog ownership. What had I missed?

As I speculated, Tarica's nurse came in. "Dr. Abel was here to tell you he's going to do everything he can to make surgery happen tomorrow, and since you weren't here, I'm supposed to tell you."

My laughter dissolved in a wash of shock. Surgery? Tomorrow? Friday? I must have been opening and shutting my mouth like a fish, because the nurse was grinning at me.

I shook my head. "But we're going home tonight."

No, we weren't. We were staying, and tomorrow, if Dr. Abel had his way, a laser would do something irreversible inside Tarica's brain.

An hour or so later, a member of the neurosurgery team came to Tarica's room with an update, which was when I learned there was another laser ablation scheduled for tomorrow. Dr. Abel had decided that since all the surgical equipment was here, why not do two surgeries back-to-back? This had never been done before, so it required getting the consent of the whole team. Not everyone had yet agreed.

Whenever I hear "never been done before," I pay attention, because I believe this is where God has stepped in. I like to think God moved the heart of Dr. Abel on our behalf.

When Dr. Abel returned in the afternoon, we discovered the lengths he had gone to for us. Not only was surgery scheduled, but it was happening first thing in the morning. After the anesthesia team had declared two back-to-back surgeries impossible, Dr. Abel had canceled the other surgery.

I felt equal parts joy and guilt. What about the other family, who had been counting on surgery tomorrow? Had we delayed relief for another child and family? My guilt was eased later when I was reassured—vaguely, because of patient privacy— that there was a good chance the other family did not feel the urgency we did.

Tarica, free of all wires, spent most of the day stringing beads and looking at books on the sofa I called my bed, refusing to return to her "stupid bed" even for her nap. I received permission to load Tarica into a wheelchair and tour the hospital, a rare treat for a child who was usually confined to her room attached to a computer by dozens of wires, under 24/7 video surveillance. She kept asking when her daddy was coming, as if she couldn't remember my last answer.

Linford hates hospitals enough that I'm relieved for his sake when he goes home, even if I'm there alone with Tarica. On normal hospital days—that is, days of waiting around for the next seizure or test or result—I'm glad he's not there, going twitchy with inaction and unanswered questions. But on days of big emotions, I miss him as badly as our daughter does.

We had agreed to surgery, but I had thought I would have more time to process this huge leap into darkness. What if surgery failed to stop the seizures? What if it not only failed but also crippled her? Or succeeded but crippled her beyond any hope of a normal life?

What if one day she would say through tears, "Why did you do this to me? Better that I only have seizures." Would this be the last day she could string beads and give me high-fives with her left hand? My head ached from all the possibilities racing around inside it. If only Dr. Abel were able to promise us surgery would be worth it.

When Linford arrived that evening, I clung to him and wished no one else were there so I could cling longer. Surgery was what we wanted, what we had prayed for. Why was I crying? This shouldn't be so hard.

Tarica delighted so thoroughly in her father's presence that she seemed to have forgotten why he was here. But after I tucked her in for the night and darkened the room, she began crying. "What if they mess up?" she whispered as I brushed tangled hair off her wet cheeks.

There was little to say in reply. I could make her no promises. What if they did laser too much or too close to something vital? Tomorrow could change her life—in beautiful or terrifying ways. We could only take it to Jesus and put our fears into His hands.

I gave up trying to sleep around four and lay awake listening to the noisy quiet of a hospital awakening. Transport came for Tarica soon after seven, and before long, she and I found ourselves outside the double doors that led to the OR unit. Her stretcher was docked in the same bay where we had waited in 2015 for her grid-removal surgery, after ten days of no seizures. Had God withheld the seizures from us then because He saw 2020 coming?

In 2015, Tarica had bounced around on the stretcher, unflapped by the grid of electrodes inside her head. At five, she did not understand what was at stake. At ten, she knew too well, and she wept quietly. She was so scared, she said.

I reached over the stretcher railing and put my arm around her as best as I could. "Do you still want to do this? If you don't, we can say no. We will not force you." I couldn't believe the words were coming out of my mouth. After everything, including canceling someone else's surgery, people would throw fits if we backed out. I held my breath as I waited for her answer.

"I still want to. I'm just scared." More tears leaked out.

"You're allowed to be scared." I handed her a tissue from the box a nurse had placed on the stretcher when he saw her crying. I grabbed one for myself. Did I tell her I was also scared? I don't remember. But I did speak of God's care and people's prayers and how she wouldn't be alone. It made us both cry even more.

Finally, she was wheeled through the double doors. I shuffled beside the stretcher, gowned and hatted and booted and masked. We passed the operating room from 2015 and wound deeper into the maze of halls until we came to another set of doors, where Dr. Abel met us.

When she saw him, Tarica started crying again. He asked her, "What are you afraid of?" His words were soft, an invitation to confide in him.

Her breath shuddered in and out as she choked out her words. "I'm afraid you'll miss it."

I flashed back to Tarica's words from last night: "What if they mess up?" I thought she was worried she would lose essential function because of the surgery. But now I saw she didn't fear they would take too much. She feared they would take too little.

Dr. Abel's eyes were gentle. "We'll do our best to get it all." No promises he cannot keep, not from Dr. Abel.

The OR looked so new I half-expected to smell drying paint. Tarica was transferred from the stretcher to a narrow, padded board. The anesthesiologists asked her about her pets as they fastened her down. She was in the middle of listing our hens' names when she lost consciousness. Someone said, "You may kiss her, Mom."

She smelled of gauze and antiseptic, not my child, but her cheek was still soft, and freckles faded by winter still paraded across her nose. As I straightened, Dr. Abel beckoned me across the room, with a warning to not brush against anything. He led me to a squat pink and white machine that had an arm jutting from it and a large screen on the far side.

"This is the robot?" I asked. It didn't look anything like the robots of my imagination.

"This is the robot." He pointed at three images of a brain. Her brain. "Here and here and here and a little bit here are the places we are going to ablate. They are in the area of her brain that helps to coordinate movement in her left leg."

Her left leg. Across the room, gowned professionals worked over a child who no longer knew she was afraid. Should I—no, I couldn't take her out of here. It was too late. She had told me triumphantly that it was okay if she needed a wheelchair after the surgery, because she knew how to use one. I had laughed, but I no longer found it funny.

What had we done?

The wall closest to us had two big sliding doors. Behind them was an MRI machine. With the help of the robot and the MRI, Dr. Abel would be able to get deep inside Tarica's brain and use a laser to burn the area where the seizures originated. A scalpel would be far less accurate, if it could even be used that deep in the brain at all. Perhaps 2015 hadn't happened because we needed 2020 technology.

It was time to go. I gingerly crossed the OR, pulling my baggy overalls against me lest I touch anything, and followed a nurse through another maze that didn't feel like the way we had come.

I met Linford in the hall outside the surgery waiting room. I shucked my suit and its accessories and dunked them into a nearby trash bin, shedding my connection to that gleaming room where our daughter lay unconscious, surrounded by strangers, save Dr. Abel.

What had we done?

The surgery could take up to seven hours. It felt as if I had seven hours of my life left, and after that—nothing. I couldn't imagine tomorrow or even this evening, because everything depended on the surgery's outcome. One way or another, good or terrible, the next seven hours would change our life. It *had* to.

Close to noon, Dr. Abel appeared and ushered Linford and me into a consultation room. The operation was over. Tarica was in the MRI for one last scan and then the bolts needed to be removed from her head. She would be taken from the OR to the ICU, where we could see her once she was awake.

As for success or failure, we wouldn't know until she woke up how much function she lost, and even then we wouldn't know if any loss would be permanent. Any seizures during the first twelve weeks post-surgery could be attributed to brain swelling from the surgery. We could draw no conclusions from what would happen next.

I felt like a clock being wound tighter and tighter. Any second now, springs and gears would snap, and time would stop. The surgery was over, the rest of our life had just begun, but here I was sitting around waiting. Perhaps this was how Linford felt every time he was in a hospital.

Early afternoon, we received word that she was finally in her ICU room. Down the hall, onto the elevator, out on the fifth floor, to the desk outside the ICU. As the unit door clunked open, it seemed as if I was watching myself in a dream. Turn left and right around a few corners, and there she was on the other side of a glass door.

She looked as if she was sleeping, but as Linford and I stopped by her bed, her eyes opened. "Is it over already?" she croaked, surprisingly alert.

"The surgery is done, and you're back in the ICU." I reached down and slid my fingers into her left hand. "Squeeze."

She squeezed.

I looked at Linford, unable to speak.

Linford moved to the foot of the bed and put his hands against the soles of her blanketed feet. "Push me away."

She pushed. With both feet.

I yanked the covers back. "Move your leg for me. Let me see it."

She moved her leg.

"Oh, Tari!" I practically fell on top of her in a hug. "You're going to be okay, sweetie." I pulled back and took her left hand again. "Squeeze again. I just can't believe it."

She squeezed. We laughed together.

I wiped away tears. "Oh, I'm so happy I could hug the whole world." And when I met a familiar nurse in the hall, I started with her.

Tarica had an unnatural curl to her left hand, and it was weaker than her right. Later we would discover that her left leg dragged when she walked. With time the weakness would likely disappear. The room pulsated with joy. Whether or not she would continue to seize, she had the use of all four limbs.

When Tarica's traumatized brain insisted on a nap, Linford and I slumped onto the sofa to replay the day. Across the room, a computer monitor flashed through a rotation of screensavers. Wash in, wash out, said one slide, promoting the practice of using hand sanitizer when you step into a patient room and when you leave. Another slide advised staff to meet people's eyes and smile. Yet another declared that this hospital and many others within the network were prepared for the new coronavirus, and for more information, go to this website.

Earlier in the week, I had gone to that website but had been interrupted before I read much. It didn't matter anymore. The coronavirus couldn't possibly affect us as much as what had taken place this day.

A week after Tarica's surgery, the neurosurgery department was shut down, along with the rest of our state.

In a world I no longer recognized, her surgery became my raft in a storm. If Dr. Abel had not insisted on surgery that Friday, we would have had to wait many weeks for elective surgeries to once again be permitted. Our shutdown would have been filled with far more stress and seizures. When surgery would have finally happened, only one parent could have accompanied Tarica to the hospital, per the hospital's new COVID-19 policy.

Not only had God seen 2020 coming, but He also had seen COVID-19 marching across the world. God knew and answered before we called. It's as if He looked at us and said, "I know how hard this has been. Let Me make this a little easier, even though you don't yet see what a gift it is."

There were still seizures during the shutdown and in the months that followed. Surgery was not a cure, but it did temper the seizures. Before surgery, the seizures were so frequent we struggled to function as a family. Afterward, we had enough space to live between the seizures, with more seizure-free days than not, even though she continued to seize at night.

We pray that someday we can win this fight with epilepsy. But whatever the future gives us, Tarica's surgery has shown me indisputably that God is in control, even when it seems He does not see our pain. In His careful arrangement of details, He demonstrated that, no matter what is coming our way, He is already preparing us to face it.

The first week of March 2020 has become my banner. It is a promise snapping in the winds of uncertainty: nothing can sweep us out of His hand.

Will This Be the Last Day?

Sandra Weaver

ON MARCH 27, 2020, I awoke with the same thought I'd had every morning for the past two weeks: *Will this be the last day of school?* Other schools across the country and around the world had already closed. As I dashed about preparing to make face masks in art class, I had no way of knowing this would indeed be our last day of school.

"Every day is a gift," I had told my students a week or so before. With restrictions tightening daily, we took the gift of school seriously. The idea of homework bothered me as I considered the possibility of not being able to return the next day. I wanted to do as much checking as I could before the students left for the day, in case something had been misunderstood. Was it worth writing up all the class stuff on the chalkboard for the next day? Should I put up a new bulletin board? How much practice should we put into a program we might never have? I made sure I used the devotional idea that had been floating around in my head.

We finally went ahead with achievement tests, even though two students were absent. We had no promise of tomorrow. After finishing the tests, we enjoyed a ball game under cloudy skies. Before heading inside for ice cream and dismissal, we paused for a group photo. "Let's all look at that cloud over there for a picture," a tenth grader randomly suggested. In the photo we look like a bunch of ballplayers intently staring at the heavens, watching for Jesus to appear in the clouds.

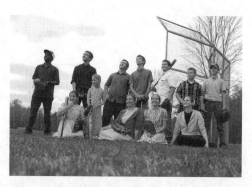

I often thought of Jesus's return to earth as we faced the reality that each school day could be our last. What if we were always this aware that today Jesus could return? What would we want to make sure we finished? What apologies and prayers would we quickly offer? I would probably drop all plans for the day to focus on reading the Bible and praying for people who aren't living right.

There were many things I failed to accomplish before school shut down: I forgot to take individual photos of my students. I didn't have that birthday party for the girls. I had wanted the whole school to take part in a true-to-life Anabaptist devotions, complete with someone coming in with handcuffs. But none of that happened. And there was so much more I wish I could have taught my students.

When Jesus comes, what will we have failed to do? Will we have neglected the important things to focus on the trivial? Which will matter more, finishing a dress late Saturday night or studying the Sunday school lesson? What about missing that youth volleyball game to stay with an elderly grandparent? Do we have a bad attitude over something that doesn't really matter? That huge disappointment we felt when our plans didn't work out will seem so pointless.

After the governor's speech at four o'clock on March 27, we were told school was closing until at least April 30. I took my students' books to each of their homes and said the dreaded goodbyes. I hastily packed at the place I had boarded for the past three years. With an aching heart, I started my hour-and-a-half drive home. I knew from experience the feelings of leaving part of my heart in a community and moving on. Only this time, it happened six weeks earlier than I had planned.

When Jesus calls us home, there will be no twisting pain of tearing up roots or letting go of the people we've learned to love. We will be Home. Our arrival will be pain-free and full of joy!

Pictorial Diary of Coronavirus in Lancaster County

Sara Nolt

RUMORS OF A deadly virus in China reached us in January. But you know how rumors are—impersonal and distant, like rumbling thunder that never produces rain. I listened to the rumors but thought a virus in Asia was unlikely to disrupt schedules in idyllic Lancaster County, Pennsylvania.

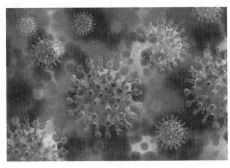

But sometimes thunder is the precursor to rain. Coronavirus came to western America in late February. It rolled across the continent, ruthlessly ravaging the elderly and immunocompromised. Unbelievably, it reached Lancaster County, that little pocket of the globe I had supposed was immune to this kind of devastation.

When the virus arrived, rumbling rumors changed from distant destruction to imminent lockdown. People rushed to stores, frantically buying necessities before a stay-at-home order was put in place. Shelves were wiped clean of pasta and peanut butter, bread and milk.

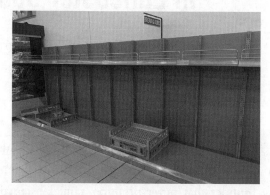

The top-selling items were toilet paper and hand sanitizer. Stores rationed the amount you could purchase. When the TP was gone, people bought paper towels until those shelves were empty too.

Online, TP prices climbed, and the date it would be shipped got pushed out a month. Or two. No one seemed to know why TP was the world's top-selling quarantine item, since COVID's symptoms were not primarily gastrointestinal.

Lancaster's stay-at-home mandate began on March 23. Nonessential businesses closed. Essential businesses limited hours, sanitized carts, and created traffic patterns in the aisles.

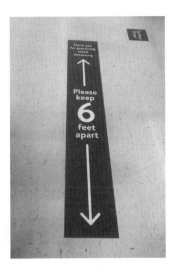

Schools closed and nearly the entire nation joined us in homeschooling.

Churches canceled in-person services. Congregants called in or watched via livestream. Toward the end of the stay-at-home order, our church had one family per week sing hymns on livestream as a way of adding worship to the living room services. My daughter illustrated that portion of the service.

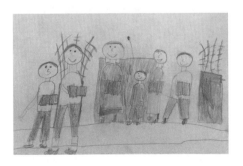

After a month of staying home, we understood the passion behind the crying preschooler who said, "The only thing open is *nothing*."

Not only were public places closed, restrictions on crowds prohibited large gatherings for weddings, funerals, and graduations. We missed the funeral of John's grandma. Only her children attended while their spouses sat in vehicles along the road, watching the burial and outdoor service from a safe distance.

And when John graduated from college in May, homemade pizza and a mailed diploma replaced traditional celebrations.

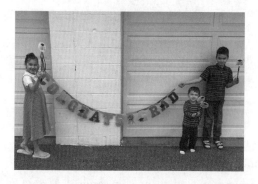

Shortly after the coronavirus reached Lancaster, masks became mandatory.

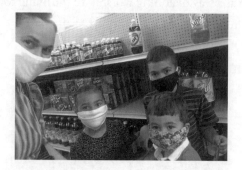

Roadside stands sprang up selling masks.

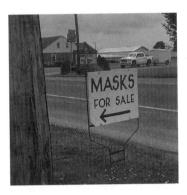

Humor helped us navigate this surreal world.

Once, a housebound family of Jug Heads stopped in long enough to add interest and humor to our evening.

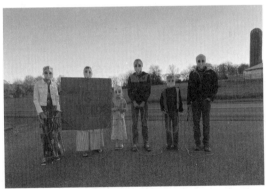

The stay-at-home order, depressing statistics, canceled plans, and interrupted life grew wearisome.

The stay-at-home order for Lancaster County was finally lifted on June 4, seventy-four days after it was put in place.

We are now in the green phase of reopening. Masks and social distancing are still required, but rumors of hope are circulating:

"The virus is weakening."

"Not as many people are dying."

"The nurse told me on July 8 that while they see a lot of positive COVID tests, there are fewer hospitalizations. Last week Lancaster General had forty COVID patients; this week there are only twenty-eight. Out of the twenty-eight, only three are intubated."

Hope. Amid the uncertainties of Life with COVID, this one thing remains unchanged.

For I am persuaded that neither life nor death nor coronavirus nor quarantine nor things present nor things to come can ever separate me from the love of God.

Unorthodox Ordination

Diane Martin

AFTER ALL THESE weeks of seeking God's will through prayer, we are finally here, I thought as I scraped the leftover tomato soup into a plastic container. *Tomorrow morning is the nomination service.* I put the soup into the fridge. Turning to my six-year-old daughter, I said, "Annika, you should be taking a bath."

By tomorrow evening we will know who is called to share the lot. My thoughts ran as fast as the dishwater running into the sink. They became a prayer as I plunged dishes into the hot, soapy water. *Lord, may Your will be done.*

"Hey, Dad, did you hear that Premier Doug Ford might restrict gathering size to two hundred fifty people?" I heard seventeen-year-old Lyndell ask. "What would we do about the ordination if that happens?"

"Hard telling," Allan replied. "In Alberta they've restricted gathering size already."

The men continued to discuss the situation, but I didn't hear. I was too busy thinking and praying. It was a ridiculous idea anyway. Whoever heard of a church gathering being limited or canceled in our country?

Our home congregation, Meadowside, had grown so large it had been divided into two districts in January 2018. The minister and deacon of Meadowside both lived in the east district, so we knew a few ordinations were ahead for those of us who made up the west district. In August 2018, a minister was ordained for Meadowside West. Our former deacon had done a good job of looking after us during the past two years, but it was time to spread out the load. We looked forward to having a full team of ministry for our district. Only God knew whom He had chosen to fill this office, and we wanted His will to be done among us.

On Sunday morning, we went to church with prayerful hearts. As I went around the circle in the church lobby greeting my dear sisters in Christ, we were all aware that changes were on the horizon for our congregation. Unknown to us, there were more changes than the ones we imagined. How little we guessed we would not gather for services at Meadowside again for three months, and that when we did congregate again, we would use hand sanitizer outside the door and try to stay six feet apart instead of greeting each other. On March 15, 2020, we greeted each other in a special way, with meaningful hand squeezes, and looked each other in the eye. None of us knew about "social distancing" back then. The love and closeness in our midst was precious. There weren't many visitors—it was just our Meadowside West "social bubble." (Except we hadn't heard of social bubbles yet either.)

We were once told that before a nomination service, it feels as if the whole congregation is in the lot. After the nomination service, several share the lot and the rest are released. Due to church growth, our family has changed home districts or been part of a new congregation a number of times in the last twenty years. Five times before, we have attended a nomination service in our home district. Always before we were released on nomination Sunday. This time the name *Allan Martin* was read along with three other names: Cleon Weber, Marcus Bauman, and Bradley Reist.

Now we are this far, was my first thought. Annika patted my arm and whispered, "They said Daddy's name!"

I had always pictured that hearing my husband's name would give me a heavy feeling, but I found it to be almost the opposite. In the past, a feeling of heaviness would settle over me when we heard who was in the lot. This time, it wasn't there. Later, I realized why: the people's prayers shift from the whole congregation to the ones who share the lot. Other times, the prayers of the congregation didn't carry us on because we were released from sharing the lot. Though the possibility of serving with my husband in the office of a deacon looked like a heavy responsibility, the prayers of the saints eased the burden.

We arrived home from church to a yard full of vehicles. It was my turn to host the youth boys, and I had told our sons to go ahead and bring their friends home as usual regardless of whether we were in the lot. Everyone needed to eat somewhere, and I knew our boys would be glad for the support of their friends. Several of Allan's sisters came too, and with their help we soon had a meal on the table. Twenty-three people gathered for dinner. Not one of us thought about social distance as we pulled up our chairs.

After the flurry of serving dinner was past, Allen's sisters took over the cleanup while Allan and I had some precious time alone. We needed to pray together again, as we had done for months—*Thy will be done, whatever it is.* In our church group, it is customary for the ministry, family, and friends to visit in the homes of those who are in the lot. This means that sometimes the husband and wife hardly have a chance to be together alone until evening, so those minutes were a special privilege. Callers started coming around two o'clock, and except for about an hour over suppertime, people surrounded us for the rest of Sunday. We appreciated each one.

A recurring theme in the conversations among our visitors was the coronavirus. Some people greeted us as usual when they arrived—shaking hands and practicing the holy kiss. Some people chose to only shake hands. Some chose to give a wave of hello and leave it at that. For the first time, I began to realize that this coronavirus was real.

"We officially got word that no American ministry will come up for the ordination," the bishop's wife said. "There is talk of closing the border, and no one wants to risk it."

An ordination without American visitors? This would certainly be unusual. It is our custom to have preachers and deacons from our sister churches in the United States help at our ordinations.

"My in-laws didn't go to church the last two Sundays," another woman said. "Large gatherings are really being discouraged."

"I heard that someone said the Mennonites would rather hold funerals than give up their socializing," someone commented.

It took a minute for me to get that. Hold funerals? Oh! Someone was suggesting we would rather have people get coronavirus and die than stay apart from each other. Surely not! Was the situation that grave?

"That isn't a very good witness," one woman exclaimed. "We need to comply with the government rulings."

When they weren't talking about coronavirus or the Spanish flu or other epidemics from the past, various callers mentioned the need to "be there" for our children. When yet another person reminded me to consider what our children might be thinking or feeling during this time, my sister-in-law Ellen said, "I have often been told that too—to be there for my children because they lost their father. So sometimes I see them sitting somewhere, alone and quiet, and I think, *Okay, I should initiate a little talk.* I sit down beside them and ask, 'What are you thinking about?' and they shrug and say, 'What's for supper?'"

Allan and I talked until late into the night. There was so much going on, so many uncertainties, and yet such peace, as we surrendered it all to our dear heavenly Father. Once more we said from our hearts, *Thy will be done.*

Work is a tonic for me, so I was glad to see Monday morning come with its regular routine of making lunches, sorting laundry, and cleaning the church shoes and suits. While the school children ate breakfast, I tried to ask some gentle questions and encourage them to talk, in the event they were thinking about something besides what was for supper. We talked about the sermon on Sunday, and how it felt to hear the bishop read Daddy's name. One of the boys said, "When he went over all the things a deacon should be, I knew our dad is all those things."

Monday passed rather quickly. We got phone calls and texts from people who hadn't dropped in on Sunday. Some of our American friends let us know they wouldn't be able to make it to the ordination, but they would remember us in prayer. Coronavirus continued to be a hot topic on the phone and in the conversations among the men in our house who followed the news. Gathering size was now officially restricted to two hundred fifty people, and one son predicted that the number would soon be down to fifty. Sports events were on hold, and movie theaters were closed. I still didn't worry about how we would proceed with the ordination. Churches were a totally different category than sports and movies.

That evening, Allan joined a teleconference with other school advisory board members about the increasing pressure to close our schools. The public schools were closed, and while the government was strongly recommending private schools follow suit, it wasn't mandatory. The board decided to keep our schools open for the time being.

"There's no point in closing our schools as long as we are still going to church," Allan told me after the meeting. "We have a much bigger group from a larger geographical area at church than we do in our small, rural schools."

It is customary for our church group to hold an examination service for the candidates on the Tuesday afternoon before the Wednesday morning ordination. When I got up on Tuesday, March 17, I didn't have plans for the forenoon. The three men went to work, and the four youngest children left for school. Shortly afterward, our electricity went off, limiting my choices about what to do. I decided to take my daily walk. I hoped I would come back to find our electricity on.

It was our son Quinton's day to take a food to school starting with the first letter of his name. On Saturday I had fried twenty quesadillas and put them in the freezer. I had actually remembered to get them out of the freezer on Monday evening, but I needed to heat them and take them to school before lunch. After I got back from my walk, the electricity was still off, so I worked at folding Monday's laundry.

Miriam called mid-morning. She and her husband were on their way in from northeastern Ontario, about six hours away, with plans to stay in the area overnight so they could attend the ordination the next morning. "We're in the Toronto area," she said, "and we just got word only fifty people will be able to attend the ordination. Is that true?"

"It might be," I said, hardly wanting to believe it. "No one has officially told me that."

When I got off the phone with Miriam, I called the hydro company. A mechanical voice informed me our electricity would probably be restored by one o'clock. It was already ten o'clock—high time to figure out another plan for heating the quesadillas.

Back to the phone I went. "Marlene, do you have your generator running?" I asked my fellow school mom. Soon I was preparing to take the quesadillas to our neighbors. The phone rang again—a different school mom.

"A teacher called," she began, "and there is no electricity at school either. Where could we get water for school?"

"I'm going to Marlene to heat my food," I told her. "I'll take pails and a water jug along. I'm sure Marlene will let us have water."

Is this really happening? I wondered as I drove down the road with my food and pails. It seemed too shambolic to be running around in frantic circles during such a solemn, soul-searching period in our lives.

Allan's morning was also chaotic. At nine thirty, the premier of Ontario had declared a State of Emergency in the province, due to the coronavirus, and ordered the closure of all private schools. Allan was in charge of keeping the rest of the advisory board posted with government updates, so he printed the orders and delivered them to a fellow board member, along with his consent to close our schools, despite the decision they had reached only last evening.

When Allan came home around eleven thirty, I wasn't there. I had gone back to Marlene to pick up the now-hot quesadillas and the water for school. As I passed our elderly, widowed neighbor's house, I turned in on impulse, to check if she needed anything. Meanwhile, when Allan discovered we had no electricity, he collected his church clothes and went back to work to use the shower there. Just before noon, Allan and I were both at school. I was wearing everyday clothes, frantically cutting quesadillas into wedges. Allan was in his suit, hauling in the water for drinking, washing, and flushing toilets. Fifteen minutes later, we were on the way to the examination services, eating the lunch our kind neighbor, Marlene, had prepared for us.

"I don't know what I planned to do this morning," I told Allan as I leaned back against the seat, "but not that."

"The chaos isn't over yet," Allan predicted. During our seven-minute drive to church, he filled me in on the latest developments. Schools would close today for at least several weeks, and no more than fifty people could legally attend the ordination. "Perhaps they'll just have the ordination while we are together this afternoon," he suggested.

The whole thing seemed so unreal. I expected to wake up any time and find it was still before nomination Sunday, and laugh at my ridiculous dream.

Allan was right. The peculiarity of this Tuesday was far from over. When we got to church, signs on the door suggested we refrain from greeting each other with a handshake or kiss of peace. The ministers' wives formed a line and walked past us four ladies who shared the lot, staying back a few feet and only greeting us verbally. Although something was missing without physical contact, there was no mistaking the care and support we were receiving. Some things are felt with the heart.

About ten minutes ahead of starting time, we were invited to take our places in the main auditorium. We followed the deacon's wife and took our appointed seats. We had never attended an examination service before, but it was evident from the beginning that this would not be a typical one. The bishop announced that social gatherings over fifty people were against the law, and we had a larger number than that. "What should we do?"

Not everyone was aware of the ruling, since it was only passed that morning, but it didn't take long for ministers and deacons to say, "We need to obey the law." The ministry from other districts were the first to get up and leave. Later, as they counted the people and realized more could stay, some couples trickled back in.

Once the gathering size had been settled, the service was opened with a song. I tried my best to pull my scattered thoughts together and concentrate on the absolutes of God instead of the absurdities of the situation. How comforting to know that God is the same yesterday, today, and forever

No coronavirus can change that. What peace soothes the soul as we surrender and say, "Have Thy way, dear Lord."

Later in the service, there was a discussion about how to proceed with the ordination. Since only fifty people would be able to attend, the service would be held at our Goshen meeting house, the only one of our church houses with a call-in phone system. Next, we needed to decide which fifty people could attend the ordination the following day. They started with deciding which of the ministry would be there.

Our home bishop, of course, and usually three other ministers and four deacons take part at an ordination service. It was decided only two ministers besides the bishop would be needed. And they would manage with only three deacons—the one who read the text would also help shuffle the books. Or should they have only two deacons shuffle the books? No, it was decided there should be three. Marcus's dad is a deacon, but normally the father of someone in the lot wouldn't help shuffle the books. This time he would.

Everyone who could fill double-duty would have to. The six ministry men would also take care of choosing and leading the songs and any ushering duties that needed to be done. What about the wives of those six men? Of course they must attend, no debate about that. That was twelve people, so thirty-eight more could attend. There were four couples in the lot, with a combined number of twenty-three children.

That's when it hit me how *few* people a group of fifty is. With the four couples in the lot, their children, and the six ministry couples, we already numbered forty-three. What about our parents? The rest of our Meadowside congregation would not be able to attend. Siblings were out of the question.

Did we all want to have our preschoolers there or would we rather leave that room for our parents? Should we count only the children school-age and up? Marcus and Brad immediately said they would rather leave their two youngest at home to make room for their parents.

I knew that age-wise, our Annika was the next in line to cut off. Did a kindergartener count for a school child? It had *not* occurred to me we might need to make such a decision. Allan's parents weren't planning to attend because of health reasons. I thought about my mom. She lives here. She is part of our family, but I knew she would be the first to say, "Oh, if there isn't room for everyone, then I don't have to go."

Allan and I communicated across the church. When asked whom we wanted to have attend, Allan replied that if our six children could come, we were satisfied to leave it at that. Mom said to me later, "If it was between Annika and me, *of course* Annika was the one to be picked."

On the way home, we stopped in at school to pick up the leftover quesadillas. The teachers were coming to grips with the fact that, suddenly, on a Tuesday afternoon in March, school had come to an abrupt end.

When we got home, Allan's sister Wilma had brought salads from the restaurant where she worked, because it had to close that day. Grandma had cooked a ham for us, perfect to eat with potato and macaroni salads. How handy, since my plan to get something into the oven for supper hadn't materialized that forenoon. God provides!

In spite of the confusion of the day, sleep came easily that evening. The peace that passeth understanding surrounded us. The thing that bothered me most was the feeling that the strange events were keeping me from realizing the solemnity of the ordination. It was a comfort to know that even this was not a secret from our great God. He knows my frame and remembers that I am dust.

We awoke soon after three o'clock on Wednesday morning. Although sleep eluded us, we continued to feel surreal peace as we shared and prayed together. My mom came over for a seven-thirty breakfast of baked oatmeal. After eating, we sang, one song being number 401 in the Christian Hymnal. "Ready to go, ready to stay..."[1] Our children are blessed with good singing voices, and I love to sing with the family. It was touching to see and hear their fervent voices. We also sang "Tomorrow in Your Hand."[2] *Help me to leave tomorrow with You, Jesus...*

My mom went to my brother David's place to listen to the ordination service. It made me feel better knowing she was with family and other church people. I felt a little guilty we could go to the ordination, when most of our fellow Meadowside congregation couldn't attend. Many of them dressed up in their Sunday black and met together in homes in groups of up to fifty, to listen to the ordination service together. The frustrating part for them was that the phone line didn't work properly. No one could listen in until an hour and fifteen minutes after the service began. At least they were connected by the time the ordination was held.

Having ministers come to an ordination from across the border is a special, long-standing custom at our ordinations,

1   Ready to Do His Will, ascribed to A. C. Palmer
2   Tomorrow In Your Hand, used by permission

but as our group of fifty people gathered on the front benches at Goshen church, it was precious to have our familiar leaders take charge of the service. I learned a new word during the ordination sermon, when the minister talked about COVID-19. Up until that day, people just referred to the coronavirus.

The atmosphere was so family-like. We thought about the verse in Matthew 18:20, "For where two or three are gathered together in my name, there am I in the midst of them." The many empty benches did not make us feel forsaken. We knew we were "compassed about with so great a cloud of witnesses." There was more support felt than what could fit into the church house.

And then the time was at hand. We knelt once more, surrendering all to God and pleading for His will to be revealed. Later I told Allan, "I had been praying for the bishop as he set the books, and for the four men to have strength for the moment, to choose the book God had planned for them, grace for the task of taking a book...but suddenly I realized I was praying for only one man anymore! I trust the other wives had the rest covered."

The lot fell on the oldest couple, Cleon and Ruth Weber. Again, our hearts said *amen* to the will of God. We felt such awe as we watched God reveal His will. After months of prayer, He allowed us to know what He had in mind. It was humbling to think of His care for poor mortals such as we.

Because the lot was found in the first book, Allan never handed his book to the bishop. I knew that the man who is ordained keeps the slip of paper with the words "The lot is cast into the lap..." but I hadn't known that each man in the lot keeps his book. On our dresser is Allan's "empty" book with a pamphlet the bishop gave him, "Called to Be a Layman." The pamphlet reminds us that every book has a calling—if not to a new place, then a calling to keep on in the place we were. It is our earnest desire to serve wherever God wants us.

In the evening our family sang "Ready to Do His Will" again, this time knowing what to expect. Allan reminded us, "We don't know what tomorrow will hold any better than we knew what today would hold, but the unknowns of an ordinary day feel more familiar."

Except we aren't sure what ordinary means anymore. Government officials talk about the "evolving" situation. That's very much how it continues to be—COVID-19 is an evolving event, and we must somehow evolve with it. What peace we have as we remember that our God is not an evolving God. He never changes! With our eyes fixed on Him and our hand in His, we go on in confident faith.

Never Out of Stock

Hertzen Kruse

SHELVES LIE BARE in the wake of frantic shopping sprees. No toilet paper. No cleaning products. No hand sanitizer. No Vitamin C. No rice or flour. Not even ice cream. Signs dot the shelves, limiting quantities and apologizing for shortages.

Shopping baskets and carts, checkout counters, and credit card machines are wiped with sanitizer—and re-wiped. And wiped again.

Smiles have gone undercover. Shoppers exchange suspicious glances and give each other wide berths.

Has kindness gone out of stock too? Is excessive sanitation killing germs *and* courtesy?

My job at a local bulk food store has provided an interesting view of society's reaction to this pandemic. I fought disgust at the way human nature glared until God showed me that my attitude was just as repulsive to Him as others' selfishness. Another person's lack of courtesy was no reason to let my own compassion fade. As I looked at the world with renewed vision, examples of kindness suddenly abounded.

On two separate occasions, young women turned to the elderly customer next in line and paid for their groceries.

A big, burly man carried a box of groceries out to a little old lady's car.

An elderly man hobbled to open the door for another customer laden with purchases.

A woman was almost out the door when she realized she had missed paying for one of her items. The customer behind her handed the checkout girl a handful of dollar bills to cover the cost.

Though some customers refused their change because they didn't want to touch it, many told us to keep it as thanks for our services.

Those customers may or may not consider themselves Christians, but they were still showing love to a fearful, hurting world. How much more should I, as a child of God, do my part to ensure that kindness and courtesy are never out of stock?

Elevators and Incubators

Kristen J. Horst

TWO MEN IN black uniforms steered the stretcher into my hospital room. How unreal. I was headed an hour and ten minutes away to Harrisburg UPMC hospital, where our first baby was probably going to be born six and a half weeks early.

The nurse popped her head in the door, phone to her chest. "Were you out of the country in the last month? They want to know."

Kraig and I looked at each other, calculating how long it had been since our visit to the Dominican Republic. "No," I answered, "it's been longer than that."

"Are they asking because of the coronavirus?" Kraig asked.

She rolled her eyes and shrugged as she turned away. "Probably." She disappeared down the hall, and soon I was wheeled to the ambulance, my IV pole tagging behind me like a tail.

I was diagnosed as severely preeclamptic; my symptoms were high blood pressure and elevated liver-enzyme levels. The liver enzymes kept rising, so two days later on Saturday, March 7, we welcomed Mitchell Kade in all his four-pound, seven-ounce manhood.

A NICU team took our crying, dark-haired boy, hooked him up to oxygen and an IV, and transferred him to a cozy incubator. Mitchell needed to learn to breathe on his own, take all his food by mouth, and regulate his temperature in the safety of the hospital's NICU.

What would we do when I was discharged? We wanted to be with our son as much as possible. On one of our visits to the NICU to see Mitchell, Britney the social worker introduced herself and offered to help us in any way she could. She told us about free lodging—at Bailey House—within walking distance of the hospital.

"Sounds great," we agreed. By Tuesday my liver-enzyme levels had dropped enough that the doctor discharged me, and we moved our luggage to a room on the second floor of Bailey House. The room contained two single beds, and we would need to share a bathroom with others, but minor inconveniences were worth it if we could be near Mitchell.

Our days settled into a routine. We walked to the hospital in the crisp morning air and took the back elevator up to floor nine. At the NICU entrance we picked up the phone.

"Hello?" the receptionist answered.

"This is the parents of Horst."

"What's his code?"

"0951."

"Come on in."

The doors swung open at her command, and we walked into the NICU, one step closer to our tiny miracle. We signed the guest book, placing our relationship to Mitchell in the blank: *Daddy, Mommy.* Next we used the foot pedal to squirt sanitizer onto our hands, smearing it to our elbows. At last we were ready to see Mitchell.

"Hi, Mitchell," we would say as we walked into his room and sanitized our hands again, just to be safe. The days drifted by as we watched Mitchell grow and helped with his "care times" every three hours. Soon the nurses let us change his diaper and check his temperature ourselves. Sometimes I held him skin-to-skin while his food pumped slowly through a feeding tube.

Every day we welcomed family and friends, plus the food they brought along. Mitchell kept growing and reaching milestones. On day four, he said goodbye to respiratory support. His bilirubin lights were dismissed on Friday, day six.

Rumblings about COVID-19 ramped up. Folks asked us if we could still have visitors. "So far, so good," we said. But then...

Saturday, March 14, we mentioned that some of our friends were planning to come that evening. The nurse told us she had heard that visitors were soon going to be denied access. "But it has to filter down through the administration," she explained. It sifted through the sieve in a few hours; at one thirty, a nurse stepped into the room.

"I'm the head nurse for this floor," she said after asking how we were. "The administration has decided to ban all visitors except parents to the NICU because of the coronavirus. Also, the receptionist will be asking you a few questions before you are allowed in the NICU."

"Okay," we said.

"We're all in this together, and we're asking for everyone's cooperation. We need to work together during this time." Her startling blue eyes made me nervous.

"When does it go into effect?" Kraig asked.

"Right now. I came to tell you first, because a nurse mentioned you were expecting visitors tonight."

Kraig and I looked at each other. That was that! No more visitors. Our friends decided to come anyway and take us out to eat, so we met them outside the hospital with some photos of Mitchell.

As we headed to Ruby Tuesday for dinner, I gazed out the window at Harrisburg. I had been whisked to the hospital in an ambulance after dark, and the three-minute walk to Bailey House had been the extent of my excursions. We crossed the Susquehanna River and passed stately homes. How ironic! Because of COVID-19, I could now enjoy a tour.

Two hours and an elevator ride later, Kraig picked up the phone to call the NICU for entrance.

"Okay, I'll need to ask you a couple of questions. Have you been out of the country in the last two weeks?"

"No."

"Have you been in contact with anyone who is under investigation for the virus?"

"No."

"Do you have any signs of upper-respiratory illness, such as fever, cough, shortness of breath?"

"No."

"Come on in."

The NICU grew quiet as only parents and staff roamed the halls. Nurses discussed COVID-19. They needed to cancel birthday parties they had planned for their children. They laughed at photos of masked people sitting in airports. "They wear them like this," one nurse said, demonstrating with his own mask. "Big gaps in the sides."

The next morning, to our surprise, the housekeeper at Bailey House stopped us as we passed through the kitchen on our way to the hospital.

"They are shutting down Bailey House because it is group housing," she said in broken English, her colorful skirt flaring around her.

"When does this take effect?" Kraig asked.

"This morning," she said. "The social worker will call you about it."

Now what? Would we still have a place to stay? We discussed the situation as we walked the familiar path to the hospital.

We once again arrived at the NICU doors. "Do you have any signs of fever or upper-respiratory illness?"

"No."

"Have you been out of the country since . . . last night?" she asked, putting a spin on the real question.

"No." Laughing, we entered the NICU.

Britney the social worker came to our rescue, arranging for us to stay at a Quality Inn for free. So on Sunday afternoon, we packed our belongings and drove to the hotel. Now we could have a private bathroom and a king-size bed; COVID-19 had granted us a luxury!

Monday—the day I had dreaded—arrived. It was time for the new daddy to return to work. Kraig dropped me off at the outside elevators, and with a lump in my throat, I watched him leave. I was alone in the huge hospital with Mitchell.

The next day, I needed to go to the hospital lab for blood work. As I walked into the main entrance of the hospital, germs seemed to assail me from all sides. What if that sick-looking man coughed coronavirus germs on me? I walked as if I considered blood work to be a rare prize I was in danger of missing. At the lab I spotted a hand-sanitizer station. Oh, great! I liberally doused my hands. At least we could go to the NICU by the back elevators, avoiding the rest of the hospital. Or so I thought.

"I have a stiff neck," I commented to Kraig as I crawled out of bed on Wednesday morning.

"Since when?"

"I just realized it in the middle of the night."

"Hope it feels better soon."

We drove through the dawn to the elevators. I hoisted the backpack to my shoulder, grabbed the satchel, and said goodbye to Kraig. As I approached the elevator room, I saw a yellow paper taped to the door. It informed me that because of COVID-19, they were asking everyone to use the main elevators inside the hospital. Oh no. Kraig had used those elevators a few times to help our visitors find the way, but I had never navigated them. I tried the door just to be sure. Locked.

A few nurses came up behind me; one used her badge on the door. It didn't budge. "What's going on?" she asked as she waved her badge several more times. "I thought nurses could use these elevators."

I straightened my shoulders and soldiered to the main hospital entrance, nurses following. Inside, everyone funneled through an interrogation checkpoint. Before, our NICU wristbands had provided us with any access we needed.

Today a young lady with a chirpy voice asked where I was going and proceeded with the three traditional questions, even though I would be asked the same things at the NICU.

She approved my entrance, and I searched for the path to the elevators. Nurses swished past in their morning rush; I followed their lead. Stepping onto the elevator, I pushed the button for floor nine. We stopped at floors four, six, and seven. At nine, the nurses rushed off as I looked around the hallway. Where was I? If only Kraig were here. I had no clue where I was going. Tears pricked my eyes and my shoulder muscles tensed as I turned left. Ahead were swinging doors. It seemed I was heading into forbidden territory. I retraced my steps and cowered in the corner, swallowing hard to get rid of the lump in my throat. Instead, it grew bigger, and a few tears escaped.

I decided to call Kraig for help.

"Hello, my dear," he said.

"Hi," I replied, working to keep the quiver out of my voice. "They won't allow us to use the outside elevators anymore, so I had to go inside, and I can't figure out where I am." I ended with a sob, and as he started asking questions, the elevator door opened, and a smiling nurse stepped out.

She paused as she noticed me. Apparently I looked more like a little lost ducky than a competent NICU mom, because she asked, "Where are you going?"

"To the NICU."

"Hey, a nurse came," I said to Kraig and ended the call.

"Oh, you're in the wrong building," the nurse explained. "This is the ninth floor, but it's pediatrics. You'll have to go back down and use the other set of elevators to go up to the maternity floor, then go to the NICU."

"Thanks. I was used to using the outside elevators."

"No problem; it's confusing." Off she went while I waited for an elevator to take me to the ground floor once again. The only way I could figure out how to get to the other set of elevators was to go back through the checkpoint.

Chirpy Voice eyed me suspiciously as I paused to ask, "Do you know which elevators to take to get to the NICU?"

"Ask at the front desk," she chirped. By now the backpack and satchel felt as if they were loaded with ball bearings instead of food and personal items for a day in the NICU. Sweat began to trickle.

I explained my dilemma to a kind-looking security guard at the front desk, and with a glance at my wristband, he showed me to the elevators. Sure enough, a purple sign above them read "NICU & MATERNITY." I pushed the button and waited and waited and waited as nurses rode up and down during a shift change.

At last the elevator arrived, and three nurses rushed in. "Is there room for me, too?" I asked. They nodded as one used her knuckle to push the button for her desired floor. I felt like a leper and shrank back into the corner.

"Where are you going?" one asked.

"To the NICU. It's the first time I've used this elevator, so I don't know where I'm going," I babbled.

"Just follow us," she said.

Relief! A nurse was willing to show me the way.

I followed them off the elevator at floor eight, where she buzzed ahead with her fellow nurses. Down the hall, around the corner, and down another long hall we went. I lagged behind and let tears cleanse my chestful of emotions. "Why?" I murmured. "Why do I have to be up here all by myself? Why do we have to have a baby in the NICU? At least Kraig will be with me tonight when we leave, so I won't have to figure out the way back down."

At last we reached the maternity ward and the doorkeeper let us in. At the nurses' station the kind nurse pointed to a set of doors. "There you go."

When the doors swung open, I walked into the elevator area. One soon came, and I pushed the button for floor nine. The elevator thumped to a stop, and there were the NICU doors.

Pertinent questions asked and answered, I walked into the NICU, a good twenty minutes after I had started my journey. Trembling, I heaved the backpack onto the sofa. It had taken me so long to arrive, I had missed Mitchell's night nurse. How disappointing! I sighed as I called Kraig to apologize for ending our call so abruptly.

Mitchell's care time arrived at eight o'clock. He appeared quite hungry and nursed well for a bit. I decided to hold him skin-to-skin for the rest of his feeding, and he slept cozily on my chest as his food entered his belly through the feeding tube.

A couple of nurses passed by in the hall, and their voices floated into Mitchell's room as they discussed someone else's trouble getting to the NICU. "Till she got up here, she was crying."

So I wasn't the only one.

Several times when I turned my head to the right, a pain knifed through my neck and shoulder. By the time I put Mitchell back in his bassinet, a steady pain throbbed in my neck. When the nurse asked if I wanted to try feeding Mitchell at his eleven o'clock care time, I declined, explaining that I had a stiff neck.

"Are you okay?" she asked.

"Yes, as long as this pain doesn't get worse."

But it did. What could I do? My mother didn't answer her phone, but my sister thought a massage might help. As we discussed the problem, which seemed to have occurred because this tense new mom was trying to learn to nurse her baby, I turned the wrong way, and the sharp pain knifed me again. I could hardly breathe.

"Ouch! It hurts so bad!"

My cry must have troubled her, because she said, "You have to find somebody to help you!"

Kraig had the same opinion and promised to pray for me as my voice broke and tears flowed.

The nurse didn't know of a massage therapist in the hospital, but she got me disposable heat packs, which helped. Mother returned my call and advised me to lie flat on my back; that helped for a short time. I called Kraig to tell him I was feeling a little better, but it turned out to be short lived. The afternoon dragged on as the pain took over my neck and shoulder and emotions. The pain caused me to tilt my head to the right. Every time the nurse came into the room, she asked if I was all right.

"All except for this pain."

Mother called again. "Shall I come up?" she asked.

"No, because you couldn't come inside the hospital; I'd have to find my way to you outside somewhere."

At times I huddled in the corner so no one would notice me crying. "'I can do all things through Christ who strengthens me,'" I told myself, but I continued to cry. I was exhausted and in such pain, and I felt so alone. But I willed myself to hold together until Kraig came.

At last my knight walked in to behold a slant-faced wife, and I carefully laid my head on his shoulder to weep out the stress. He gave me a reassuring squeeze.

Pain shot through my neck. "Ouch!"

"I'm sorry!"

"It's okay. It just hurts so bad! I tried to be brave, but it was so hard."

"I know. My poor honey. I'm going to take off work tomorrow so I can stay with you."

A great weight rolled away when Kraig came, but the pain remained, so we said good night to Mitchell and left for the hotel. I crawled gingerly into bed while Kraig went to Walmart for a heat pack.

The next morning the pain was less, but I still needed to tilt my head to the side for relief. This time our journey to the NICU progressed smoothly.

That day Mitchell was twelve days old and had reached an important milestone. The lid to his bed was raised high. "Can he regulate his temperature himself?"

"Yes," the nurse said. "He was keeping toasty, so we popped his top." Now he just needed to learn to take all his food by mouth.

By that afternoon my pain was increasing again, so the nurse snagged an occupational therapist to see what she thought. She said the sharp pain was my muscle spasming. She recommended ibuprofen, heat, and a neck pillow to take the weight of my head off my neck. Kraig ran to the pharmacy for a pillow. Was I imagining it, or did using the pillow take away some of the pain?

The next morning, I knew. The piercing pain had been reduced to a rusty ache. Kraig had decided to take off work again, so we enjoyed the day together. Everywhere we went, we were reminded of the coronavirus. The screen in the cafeteria advised us to wash our hands for twenty seconds, and gave rules for those visiting the hospital. Even the touch screen on the vending machine stopped boasting about delicious snacks, and instead shared precautions about the virus. We touched as few surfaces as possible in the elevators and sanitized the table before we ate.

"Just got a tickle in my throat," a nurse explained after she coughed. Kraig tried to decide if his throat was sore or if he had an allergy. My mother gave us something new to worry about when she reported that my cousin and his wife were sick and had been tested for COVID-19. They had visited us last week, less than fourteen days ago. What if we had gotten the virus from them? Several days later the tests came back negative.

We were chatting with a nurse about how we thought the forbidden outside elevator seemed less germy, and she explained why they had stopped using it. Patients other than the NICU babies could have only one visitor, but people were disregarding the rules and sneaking in by the back elevator.

The hospital across the river had a case, but as far as we could tell, Harrisburg was still clear. We hoped to take Mitchell home before things got worse, but the coronavirus seemed to be closing in on us.

On Saturday Mitchell drank a whole bottle, and he kept gradually drinking more during his feedings. "I'm not sick," a nurse explained that morning. "Nurses are required to wear masks in the patients' rooms." The cleaning crew began to mop the floor with Clorox.

The next development appeared during the daily rounds. Dr. Anwar explained that if parents wanted to hear the daily report, they needed to come to the door, because the doctor wasn't going inside the patient's room unless it was necessary. Two NICU doctors, a nutritionist, a medical scribe, a social worker, and a few unidentified persons made up the group that listened to the report for each child.

A couple of days later, only the doctors did rounds. A few days after that, the doctors stayed in their offices and video-conferenced the rounds.

Meanwhile, Mitchell worked at growing. On Monday, March 23, he weighed five pounds, three and a half ounces. He nursed his first full feeding.

On Tuesday the doctor decided to only let him nurse, to see if he was eating enough to gain weight. I met up with another NICU mom and dad in the cafeteria. They hoped to take their girl home the next day. We talked about how we wished to get out of the hospital, away from all the germs, and laughed at how finicky we were about sanitizing. "I even wipe off the bottoms of my shoes," the dad said, lifting his white-striped sneaker to demonstrate.

As we parted ways, I wondered when we would get to take Mitchell home. We hoped to leave by the end of the week, but the doctor would make no promises. He said, "It's up to Mitchell."

Just like that, Mitchell took all his foods by mouth for twenty-four hours. On Wednesday morning, they removed his feeding tube. He needed to keep drinking enough for another twenty-four hours and gain weight as well. He passed his car-seat test and his hearing test.

Thursday morning on March 26, we awoke at six o'clock, and I called the NICU to see how Mitchell had done overnight. "He behaved like a perfect gentleman," the nurse said. "Come on over. The doctors already saw him, and the plan is still to go home today!"

Thank you, God! We packed our bags and took one last drive to the hospital. One last questioning session. One last sanitizing. I wanted to give the nurse a big hug, because as happy as she was about Mitchell's discharge, I could see sadness in her face as well. She had taken care of him more than most of the others had and had fussed over him. But because of "what's going on right now," we simply said goodbye and walked out with our precious little five-pound, seven-ounce man. No crowd of nurses, such as I had seen before the lockdown, celebrated our launch into the real world of parenthood.

After nineteen days in the NICU, we headed home at last, where we hunkered down to shelter Mitchell from the coronavirus. What would have been different about our experience if the world hadn't been terrorized by this sickness? We are so thankful that the God Who watched the virus touch His image-bearers also gave us the grace we needed for the elevators as we watched Mitchell grow in his incubator.

When the Labors Increase

Phyllis Eby

I SAVORED THE quiet as I cuddled my two-and-a-half-week-old son. All too soon, the stillness would evaporate as the school children arrived and woke the two preschoolers, but for now I could soak up his sweetness undisturbed.

My mind returned to the perplexities I'd been mulling over lately. How were we going to manage after the maid left on Wednesday? How would a newborn baby's schedule mesh with the unrelenting demands of a school schedule? The Kuhns's offer to pick up the school children at the halfway point, where our routes intersected, would help immensely. But how would we eat breakfast, have family worship, comb hair, *and* feed the baby by eight o'clock every morning? And what about laundry days? Obviously, thousands of other moms have managed such hurdles through the years, but this was our first baby since we had children in school, and my first time to figure it out.

I kissed the tiny man in my arms. Whatever the challenges of the next weeks, I was determined to enjoy little Marcus to the full. The advent of my last baby had been crammed with packing and preparations to move to Arizona. I'd felt as if I'd been robbed of his babyhood, and I certainly didn't want that to happen again. After the difficulties of childbearing at forty, this baby felt like an especially precious gift, one I wanted to savor.

Ah, there was the clank of the gate chain. I peeked through the blind and saw Heidi swinging the gate open. Seconds later, Theodore bounced into the house and shattered my shell of calm with his announcement. "My book bag is heavy, because I have all my books in it."

I blinked at him. "What?"

"My book bag has all my books in it!" he repeated gleefully. "No school for two weeks!"

Heidi joined him in prancing and chanting, "Two weeks of vacation!" I glanced at Lucinda, my maid, and read the confirmation in her look of mixed sympathy and amusement.

I sent the children off to change clothes and sought to steady my reeling mind. Sure, we had been hearing about the new coronavirus and how it had shut down a whole province of China. Yes, I'd read of the concern over rising numbers of cases and deaths in the United States, and we heard of a State of Emergency being declared, with recommendations to postpone or cancel meetings of more than fifty people. We'd been amused at how a little virus could shut down sports and political events in this modern year of 2020. But my mind, preoccupied with my baby, had failed to absorb the idea that our quiet lives, our tiny private school in the deserts of Arizona, could be affected by the panic.

Numbly, I told Lucinda what snacks to give the children, listened to the afternoon hubbub, and gave directions for chores. My mental gears alternately spun and stalled as I tried to envision how I could teach a second grader and a first grader, plus care for two preschoolers and a newborn. Tears came as I read an email from the school board chairman later that afternoon. "If any family begins to feel overwhelmed with the extra load this puts on them, please do not hesitate to ask for help. Wendell's, you have a baby in the home, and your maid is leaving in a few days. Don't quietly allow yourselves to become too stressed. Help is available."

I muddled through the evening, barely entering into the children's chatter. It was nearly bedtime before I was able to start making logical plans. If we were going to homeschool, the children would need a place dedicated to doing their school work. The office would be ideal, but how could that work? Wendell's desk wasn't an option. My sewing corner? I scooped sewing projects into a box, set the sewing machine aside, and closed the sewing table. That would make a desk for Heidi. For Theodore, I set up a card table.

If we were to come anywhere close to managing this, we would need to keep to a schedule, so we were up at our normal early hour. Lucinda went ahead with the laundry and ironing while I got the children started on dishes. "Having you at home makes more work for Mama," I told them, "so you're going to have to help with her work." Three-year-old Nathaniel was delighted to become table-clearer, while Theodore was promoted to breakfast-dishwasher. They kept at their work well, and we were ready to take our places in the office before eight thirty.

I parked myself at Wendell's desk, where I could feed the baby, answer questions, and keep an eye on Michael and Nathaniel through the curtained doorway. Spurred by the novelty of the situation, the children worked methodically through their lists of assignments. They were nearly finished by lunchtime. Recess time gave them all a chance to play outside while I caught my breath inside.

Nap time, however, was a disaster. Marcus wouldn't settle, and neither would Nathaniel. When Nathaniel finally went to sleep, the older children came romping into the house. They were warned to keep quiet, and I was finally able to rest a bit, determining we would need to find a better way to do this in the future. After naps, Miss Lillian stopped by to check the children's work and give the next day's assignments.

We had survived the first day. Lucinda declared it had gone well. I refrained from reminding her she was still here to help and didn't bother explaining the mental and emotional fatigue accompanying the endeavor.

The next morning at six o'clock, Lucinda departed, and we plunged into homeschooling without her. We got through our day without a lot of difficulty, but that night brought new complications. Theodore woke in the middle of the night, crying and coughing a tight, croupy cough. Cough syrup, chest rub, a rice pillow, and bathroom steam eventually helped him loosen up enough to sleep, and we went back to bed. Wendell lay awake for a while, worrying. At this point, we knew next to nothing about the new illness, except that it included flu- and cold-like symptoms. Wendell had heard of one coronavirus victim mentioning tightness in the chest. Was this just a cold, or was it…?

In the morning, Wendell texted his supervisor, letting him know about the sick children. He headed off but called me after a while to let me know that the supervisor had told him to stay home!

Wendell worked at his desk for most of the next week and a half, brainstorming a revision project for Lamp and Light. I shifted my chair to the doorway, and we kept on going.

Wendell's presence was a big help. He made runs to the grocery store (more frequent and more complicated because of empty shelves at the store), took charge of an occasional nap-time so I could rest longer, and kept little boys occupied outside.

We were enjoying a lazy Saturday when we received an email from the school board chairman. School would be closed for another two weeks, until April 13, and we would keep on with the current plan. Another three weeks, at least, of this? We needed to come up with something to keep up the children's interest. I started brainstorming…Earn pennies to buy chicks? Start digging up soil and get horse manure from the neighbor to plant a garden?

Wendell and I decided to try a garden. It was late for a spring garden for southern Arizona, and we knew next to nothing about gardening in this environment. But here was our chance to learn. Wendell borrowed a tiller and hauled in two pickup loads of manure, while I sorted through the stash of old seeds in the freezer. We made rows and hills and dropped in seeds in the little twenty-five-by-thirty-foot plot that resulted. Would they grow?

On Monday, we started a penny collection in a little metal bucket. The children earned pennies with neat writing, good grades, and work done by lunchtime, so that each assignment could add several pennies. We talked about what we would buy with the money earned. The children were enthusiastic about chicks, and the incentive plan worked well—so well, in fact, that each day became a race to see who could finish their work first. I sighed over the intensity of their competition and the daily tears shed by the loser (or whoever thought they might lose).

We were beginning to find our stride. After our morning chores were done, we would all meet in the office, where Michael and Nathaniel helped practice Bible memory before running off to play. After Heidi and Theodore started on their work, I retired to the living room recliner, where I could both see into the office and oversee the little boys. I soon learned to flip flashcards and feed the baby at the same time. Michael and Nathaniel enjoyed listening to reading stories and social studies lessons. By earnest effort, the day's assignments were usually completed by lunch, and the afternoon was free for naps and quiet play. By the time we did schoolwork, fixed meals (partly from the abundance Lucinda had left in the freezer), fed the baby, and took naps, there was little time, energy, or brain power left for anything else. But those were the most important things, and they were getting done.

We did find time for a few extra-curricular activities. At recess time one morning, I tucked Marcus into a baby carrier, and we all walked the half mile to the mailbox. Another day we made butter with a gallon of free cream. I gave each child a jar partially filled with cream, and they sat in a row on the floor, rolling the jars back and forth on their laps. It took nearly half an hour until big yellow lumps appeared. The children were all delighted with the process, drinks of cool buttermilk, and the taste of fresh butter on homemade bread.

Then there was the memorable day when we were so low on drinking water that we couldn't wait until Wendell filled jugs on his way home from work. I decided we could use a diversion, so at first recess, we loaded everyone in the van and headed for the gas station in Eloy. Marcus wasn't much impressed with the new activity, but everyone else was delighted. It was the first time in three weeks for most of us to venture beyond the mailbox.

The seven boring, straight-as-a-bowshot miles became more interesting as we examined the progress in alfalfa and cotton fields. While I filled jugs, the children stayed in the van and watched the steady stream of traffic and a passing train. In spite (or perhaps because) of the longer-than-usual recess, the children worked diligently and finished before lunch.

One Saturday morning brought a special treat—a socially-distanced surprise birthday party for Miss Lillian, at her boarding place. We set up chairs in little groups on and around the front porch, where we enjoyed punch and cupcakes and gave our gifts. Heidi and Theodore were thrilled to give the little pillows they had embroidered in their afternoon quiet times and which I had hastily pieced together. Afterward the groups reorganized, so moms and children could visit better, while still distanced. That was so refreshing for all of us, especially as we saw the children enjoying their friends.

I had to learn a few things about taking care of myself. I tried to handle one of those early laundry days alone. We worked at it and eventually got everything on the line, and then taken down and folded. I thought we were handling it well, but by evening I was shedding tears. The mental stress of trying to keep everyone happy and occupied, of figuring out what the baby's cries meant, getting some work done—by either drafting my helpers or by doing it myself—and listening intelligently to my husband's cogitations on his potentially changing jobs, was wearing. Lesson learned—ask for help! Suzi was glad to come hang laundry and mop floors until the stay-at-home order was issued.

Our church family loaded us with blessings during those weeks. The fellow minister's wife sent a weekly gift of food. The newlywed sister dropped off a casserole one day and a plate of cookies on another. Another family sent a plate of doughnuts. The local grandma patched a bagful of little boys' pants. When six-week-old Marcus's flailing hands pulled a bowl of hot soup over himself, a kind mother came over to help me evaluate whether he was burned. She helped me wrap one small spot. The school board chairman kept checking with us to make sure we were surviving. We knew that the prayers of all were making a difference in my ability to calmly keep on.

Seeing Miss Lillian's smiling face each day was another great blessing. She stopped in to pick up books to check. She would stop by again later to drop the books off and to practice flash-cards with the children. The children enjoyed the daily contact with someone they loved, and I was glad for a few minutes of conversation each day with another adult. One afternoon Miss Lillian stayed to help the children with puzzles. Another day she surprised me with a lovely lavender and yellow bouquet. Miss Lillian played mail-lady, delivering items between school friends.

Several songs strengthened my soul during this time, especially the song "He Giveth More Grace." The second verse encouraged me as I went about my work.

> When we have exhausted our store of endurance,
>> When our strength has failed ere the day is half done,
> When we reach the end of our hoarded resources,
>> Our Father's full giving is only begun.[3]

An unexpected blessing of homeschooling was seeing the children learn responsibility as they took their turns washing dishes, hanging up clothes, and digging weeds. They also had more time to enjoy their new brother. And by joining in our Bible memory time, the little boys were learning verses I wouldn't have thought of teaching them.

After a few weeks, I wrote to a caring friend who had inquired about my well-being:

> When I step back and look at what's going on in my life, I'm amazed I'm not more stressed out. My only answer is that God must be answering someone's fervent prayers on my behalf. Oh yes, we're intensely busy. Mom is needed by five children at once. The work is never done, and the house is never as clean as I would like it to be. I fall into bed utterly weary (and aching all over, now that we've been working at digging weeds).

3   Annie Johnson Flint, "He Giveth More Grace"

And yet, emotionally and physically, I'm doing well. Somehow—the grace of God, undoubtedly—I'm able to swing with it. I feel at rest, in spite of the intensity of life, as I haven't at many other points in my life.

And what of my fears that I would not find time to enjoy my sweet baby? After the first week of homeschooling I wrote:

We dearly love the wee man who has come to live at our house! The children all delight to hold him, in their different ways. Heidi thought herself greatly deprived not to be able to hold him while she had a cold this week. Theodore doesn't ask to hold him, but he glows when he's given the chance. Michael likes to hold baby, but his turns don't last long, because "he's so heavy." And Nathaniel loves long turns with baby every chance he gets! He still thanks God, in every bedtime prayer, "that we have a new baby and his name is Marcus Valente Eby." Mama could just hold him by the hour and cover his sweet face with kisses. Daddy hugs him and urges him to grow. As the weeks passed, we found even that blessing—the time to enjoy our little one—given with the grace for each day.

And when word came that school at home would continue, first until the end of April, and then until the school year was over, it was no shock, and we knew we could keep on. The children accepted the news without tears, and life continued.

And now it is six months later. The long vacation is finally over; exuberant children have rejoined their classmates at school. The six-month-old is learning the fun of school runs. Parental gratitude for God's gift of Christian schools and good teachers is deeper than ever before. And each day gives new opportunities to experience the Father's full giving of grace.

COVID Daze

Sarah J. Martin

"EVERYBODY IS WRITING about the coronavirus," I said, "so I'm not going to." But I forgot to write *toilet paper* on my shopping list one week in mid-March, so now I have a story to tell.

The first indication that my forgetfulness might have been a huge mistake was a picture one of our church brethren showed us of the bare toilet-paper shelves at our local Foodland. The next day we went to the city. Edward dropped me off at Value Village while he went to No Frills to get some paper towels for church.

"Maybe you should get some toilet paper while you're there anyway," I said as I hopped out, "in case Walmart doesn't have any."

When Edward returned, there was only one box in the back of the van. It wasn't toilet paper.

At Walmart, Edward strode off in search of toilet paper while I collected new splash pants for the younger children to wear on rainy days. Then I went to the vitamin shelves, where I met an empty-handed Edward.

A store employee walked by. As I searched for vitamin D, which our children take regularly, Edward asked the lady, "Am I seeing right, that you don't have any toilet paper?"

"Yeah," she said, shaking her head in disbelief. "People are buying stuff like crazy, and then there's none left for the ones who really need it."

There was no vitamin D—or hand sanitizer. A quick check at Giant Tiger yielded the same results.

The next day I counted toilet-paper rolls. Among the three bathrooms, we had enough to last about a week. Surely, surely by then some stores would have restocked. We could wait. It wasn't an emergency. And if worse came to worst, I knew where the old phone book was.

I went to town for a few groceries that day, and though I looked out the corner of my eye—pretending I wasn't looking—I saw only empty shelves in the paper-products aisle. Rice and pasta were nearly out of stock, and so were frozen vegetables. It felt unreal. This was happening to us?

Meanwhile, I heard stories about shoppers lining up outside the grocery store in town, waiting for opening time so they could heap their carts in a frenzy and amass enough to last far longer than two weeks. We heard of one man who bought all the toilet paper from the main grocery stores within a forty-mile radius. Panic buying?

A customer at the mill told Edward about her experience at Costco. After passing empty toilet-paper pallets, she spied a man with a cart piled high with packages of toilet paper. Though he was on his phone, she said, "Hey, sir, I'll buy just one of those packages from you for thirty dollars. Like, I really need it."

He gave her a careless glance over his shoulder, saying, "I've got bigger problems right now."

O Canada, what are you coming to? Where is your boast of generosity and respect for all?

A few days later, as our hygienic-tissue supply dwindled, I decided to try a different tactic. I could spare myself a fruitless trip to town by calling No Frills beforehand.

The automated message warned me that due to the high volume of products they carry, they could not provide availability information for all items, and they were sorry for any inconvenience this might cause.

Surely for something as important as toilet paper they will know, I thought, and pressed "2" for service in English.

While I listened to the on-hold music, I folded wash and cleaned up the kitchen. Now and then, a mechanical voice interrupted the music: "We are sorry for any inconvenience. One of our *friendly* and *respectful* service representatives will be with you soon."

At last a friendly girl actualized on the other end. To her friendly greeting (so far, so good) I said, "I'm just wondering if you have toilet paper in stock right now?"

"Which location?"

"Bancroft."

"Please wait while I find out for you, okay?"

"Sure, no problem." (Except for the little problem of needing toilet paper.)

I waited some minutes longer before the friendly voice returned. "Uh, I'm sorry, but we can't give accurate information about the availability of products, so..."

I assured her I understood.

So much for that. All that time just to find out I couldn't find out ahead of time.

Later that day, Edward and I planned to go to the bank and then to the machine shop for a planer profile he needed. He stopped at the laundry-room door on his way to wash up. "Do you think you could call ahead and find out if they have—"

I didn't let him finish. "I tried. They can't tell."

"Well, then we'll just go see." He grinned and walked on.

We did "go see." I messaged home partway through our time away, to assure the children we were doing fine, but we were stopping at most of the stores in town, which might have been an exaggeration.

I had a plan for what I would do at No Frills. The toilet-paper shelves were still empty, as we had expected. When I got to the checkout line with the groceries we did find, I asked the cashier, "Would you have an idea when another shipment of toilet paper will be in? We're a family of nine, and we actually *need* some."

She rolled her eyes, looking both sympathetic and annoyed. "I wish people would just calm down. It's been crazy. There was still stuff on the shelves when I got here at four, but yeah, it's gone by now. There is a truck here, but I don't know what's on it. I keep hoping it's TP, but I don't know."

"Is there such a thing as reserving some?" I asked hesitantly.

She shrugged. "I don't know that they do that. Your best option is probably to come back tomorrow and check."

Somewhat disgruntled, we agreed. What else could we do? Maybe if they had it until four o'clock, just maybe the frenzy was cooling some. Maybe we stood a chance, one of these times.

The next morning shortly before eight, I said to my oldest son, "Edward Dale, if you would go now, you'd get to No Frills right after it opens, and you could check if there's toilet paper on the shelves."

He lowered his brow; he doesn't like shopping.

"Heather can go along," I suggested. "She won't mind."

Meanwhile I sent a message to Brenda, our next-door neighbor who was currently in Greece: "Do you have toilet paper we can borrow if No Frills doesn't get any on time?"

At first she didn't realize I was serious, but she said they did have some in their house.

"I'll see what the children find out in town," I told her. And I thought, *My children are out foraging for toilet paper. I can't believe we've stooped to this. Was my message equivalent to begging?*

The children checked No Frills and Foodland, but came home empty-handed. By now I had no hopes left to be dashed. We meant to go out later in the day and check again, but we forgot. Maybe we despaired that the stores would ever have it; maybe we became complacent because we knew the neighbors did.

On Thursday I looked at the No Frills flyer. "Hey! They have toilet paper on sale." I opened my eyes wide and pointed at the picture in front of me. "It's $9.88 for a big package."

Edward raised his eyebrows. "Well, I need to drop off the pickup at Abe's for the seat covers. Shall we go to town and see? We'll be halfway there anyway."

A part of me doubted it would be worth it, but I agreed. After leaving the pickup in the mechanic's yard, Edward joined me in the van.

I craned my neck as we pulled into the empty parking lot at the store. "I can almost see it in there," I said hopefully. He dropped me off at the door.

I had both hoped and spoken too soon. Though it was still half an hour before the store's regular closing time, the doors were locked. I read the paper sign taped to the door: "In our flyer for March 19–26, we advertised Royale bathroom tissue, 30-roll package, for $9.88. Due to unforeseen reasons, the shipment has been delayed." I sniffed. I wondered how long it had taken them to figure out that delicate wording.

I got back in the van beside Edward. "The store is closed, and anyway, 'due to unforeseen reasons, the shipment has been delayed.'" Did I sneer?

When Edward went to the bank on Saturday, he stopped in one more time, just in case.

A truck was there, but it had not yet been unloaded. This time, Edward talked with an acquaintance who works at the store. She promised to call us as soon as they had toilet paper on the shelf. At the time of this writing, we are still waiting for the call. She's probably too busy guarding the TP pallet.

But what is a scant supply of toilet paper compared to the sickness and death some families face? When men and supply chains fail, we can continue to trust God, whose Word says, "I have been young, and now am old; yet have I not seen the righteous forsaken, nor his seed begging bread" (Psalm 37:25).

Wondering, Working, Waiting

Jessica Yoder

AUGUST 27, 2019

A week of school is behind us and I'm yet in awe. I relish this sense of accomplishment, knowing the school year has kicked off so well. A cynical sliver of me raises eyebrows and says, "Just wait." But the hope in me shakes a joyful fist, wherein is clutched the relationships I've built with my students.

Yes, hope. Because this is going to be a good year. Because we have so, so much to grow on from the last twelve months. Because we sought to plant the seed, and because God watered. And because He is already granting us glimpses of the fruit.

Because of this, we hope.

It's the kind of hope that raises its eyes above it all and sees the heart of a loving Father, gracing each moment with His wisdom and patience and tender care. Dousing each day with His faithfulness and goodness. Gifting each day with His glory, if we but raise our eyes beyond the horizon of the daily.

The kind of hope that energizes. Fills. Awes.

And when hope and awe keep in step, there is no telling what God will do.

When I tapped those words out one evening in northeast Los Angeles, little did I know how that hope would be tested, tugged at, and ached over in the next months. Our thriving school world came to a stunning halt as the haze of COVID-19 spread over our city and world. Unclarity settled in. What was going on? How were we to plan for next week--and the rest of the year?

In its three years of life, LA ROAD[4] Christian School has proved to be as much a family as a school. Birthed under the vision of Benji and Maria Beiler, LARCS grew into more than a place to learn English and long division; it grew out of a need for both parent and student discipleship. Benji and Maria's

---

4   Los Angeles Real-Life Opportunities and Discipleship

neighbor, recently immigrated from Mexico, met Jesus at LA ROAD Fellowship's summer Evening Bible Camp. Her heart's cry was for her children not to need to attend public school. Grasping giant faith in one hand and a shoestring budget in the other, Benji and Maria steered the tiny school of three with courageous Miss Lillian as the teacher.

This is where academics met parent and student discipleship.

In the next two years, we grew to nine students and four teachers—Mr. Brendon, Miss Ruthann, Miss Cindy, and me. Our little flock reflects the cultural beauty of Los Angeles, since most of our students hold Hispanic heritage. Parent-teacher conferences involve more Spanish than English, no lunch is complete without the glass bottle of Valentina chili sauce, and Takis chips are better rewards than candy. The joys and challenges of our diversity mingle grace and beauty, reflecting the One who brought it all together.

We are a school. But we are a school fueled by relationships, both with each other and with God. So many moments of our days weave in God's truth, whether it is penciled in the lesson plans, or whether attitudes, tears, or frustrations call for a minute of mentoring. As teachers, we care about adverbs and planets and the difference between wigwams and teepees. Yet, it's not the mere transmission of knowledge that fuels us. The call to care and invest in these precious relationships energizes us to unlock our gray stucco building every morning.

That last day of school began like most other days. We teachers met for our normal prayer time and meeting at seven o'clock, and our nine students soon arrived—in their pajamas, as our February Fun Days had spilled over into March.

We knew there was to be a meeting that morning, Friday, March 13, to determine the Los Angeles Unified School District's plan for COVID concerns. Although we are a private school, we follow the LAUSD schedule for the sake of consistency and simplicity. We knew school could be canceled, yet the announcement that campuses were closing for the next two weeks—and possibly longer—still stunned us. Education had to continue, of course, but no one seemed to know the rules because rules hardly existed.

As a teacher team, we had a host of decisions to make. As a small school, did we have to follow suit? Couldn't we simply "be careful" and quietly carry on with studies on busy Eagle Rock Boulevard? But what would that communicate to our patrons and the world around us?

Two weekends before, our teacher team had walked through several days of intense training on personalities, teamwork, and vision. As we sat around the Beilers' living room, we had learned anew how to embrace our God-given personality differences, communicate honestly, and journey together toward mutual goals. Now, two weeks later, we sat around a kitchen table with a few new tools to help us weld a plan we'd never expected to craft. For the sake of our testimony as a school, we opted to abide by the LAUSD plan.

Never would we have guessed, that rainy last day of normal school, that it was to be the first of many days teaching pajama-clad students.

Our carefully crafted kitchen-table plan? It didn't work.

That plan included a three-day school week. After shuffling plans among the teachers, we began again the following Wednesday. Miss Cindy and I met with four siblings at school. Miss Ruthann went to the Beiler household, and Mr. Brendon traveled to meet two other students. It was clunky, at best, but it kept education going for two whole days.

Then California ordered all nonessential businesses and interaction to shut down.

In those first few weeks, God gently handed His truth and steadiness to me in fresh ways, which were reflected in my journaling.

March 18

> When I shared from Psalm 46 for devotions on our first day of "homeschool," my vision was to remind four young hearts that despite change, fear, and uncertainty, God is our refuge. He is our rock, and He will not change. Nayeli added that we have God as our refuge living in our hearts—a soul-stilling, intimate image I'd never quite considered.
>
> What I didn't realize this Tuesday, when I so tidily shared those facts, was how soon I'd desperately need the reminder, too.
>
> Six days ago, life was normal. Life was beautifully unpredictable in our small school. I knew

who I was as a teacher and what I was supposed to do. I had plans and dreams and goals and not enough time to accomplish them. I built my life around loving my school family.

Now it's today, and life is starkly unpredictable. Our tiny school building is dark and cold with lonely textbooks opened to "tomorrow's lesson." Those dreams and goals? Now I have time to plan them, but the spark flickers. I love my school family, but now with the sharp pang of change and separation.

Last night as these realities settled in afresh, again I turned to Psalm 46—this time not to neatly package truth for young hearts but to calm my own. Ever notice the turmoil in this psalm? Mountains tremble and slide into the sea, waters roar, nations rage, kingdoms totter, and the earth melts. Just a few things to turn life upside down. Yet God speaks through the unrest: *Be still, and know that I am God. I will be exalted.* Be still? God, I understand You being exalted, because that's what You do. You have ways of glorifying Yourself in the midst of earthly upheaval. But You want ME to be STILL when my whole minute existence flips over?

And in the silence, He speaks.

Be still, because I still am.

Still my rock, my safe place,

shelter of my heart.

Even Nayeli knew that.

The next Monday, we met to plan online school.

This is where academics and discipleship met technology. Now instead of schedules revolving around classrooms and the bell, our schedule orbited available devices, solid Wi-Fi, and semi-quiet workplaces for the students. We needed to weave practicality, feasibility, parental preference, and our grappling minds into a workable plan for all.

We were four teachers with an assortment of experience and training, but nothing in all our seminars or tidy college courses had equipped us for online school on the fly. Live classes, teacher-taught videos, or Abeka streaming? What about homework? And grading? What subjects should we focus on, and what did we have to let go? We settled on a blend of teaching formats built around the most critical classes: English, math, history, and science. These conversations stretched us as we navigated honesty, preferences, ideals, and sacrifice.

Again we shuffled lessons, this time grouping materials by family. The next day, we delivered baskets of books and lesson-filled binders to each household, beginning a new biweekly rhythm. We also helped each family set up Google Duo in preparation for classes the next day.

At 8:27 a.m. on Wednesday, March 25, the distinctive Duo ring beckoned each family for devotions, and our first day of online school hit the screen.

Although the future of LARCS occupied most of my thoughts, our church community and neighborhood vied for attention, too. Everyone was touched in some way, and everyone had unprecedented decisions to make. Single moms in our church

needed to wrestle with work schedules—if they still had a job—
and childcare for their now-homebound children. Choice Books
staff needed to weigh their servicing options, which included
many pharmacies and hospitals. Parents needed to wisely guide
their children through the unexpected changes and decide what
physically protecting their family looked like in the midst of it all.

My heart curled up.

Everything I loved about life essentially disappeared or was
reduced to a blurry tile on a screen. In those first few weeks,
I wiped a shocking number of tears, which often sprang up
without warning or permission. Even though I lived with two
others who also loved and missed our students, I grew ashamed
of my inability to gracefully handle this change.

Now was the time to study, but I didn't have the heart to
open that language arts book I'd been eagerly devouring just
a few weeks earlier. Even thought I now had time to shorten
my book stack, I didn't feel like reading. Now was the time to
tackle new sewing projects—I even bought fabric from a friend
to prepare—but my inspiration fizzled, and I piled the fabric
away in the closet.

I felt guilty. I was healthy, and so were my friends and family.
In the weeks of uncharacteristic gloom and rain at the beginning
of Safer at Home, I had a safe, cozy home to stay in. I didn't have
to depend on free boxes of food handed out in school parking lots.
Our school had the technology to stay connected, and unlike
hundreds of teachers in our city whose students never logged in
for classes, we still had relationships with our students. There was
no justifiable reason to complain. I was just sad.

April 2020

Oh, Father,

It's only been a few weeks, and yet there's so much to miss.

I want to hear them sing their lungs out during devotions, to watch their eager faces as they await who the Player of the Week will be. I want to hear them squawk for the Valentina at lunchtime, to hear their squeaky "Miss!" on the playground. I want to glimpse their smiles of quiet pride when they finish that challenging assignment or receive a well-deserved compliment. I want to hear their questions in the hallway between classes or after school as they process life and the God Who gave it to them.

Lord, I'm not an online teacher. I don't want to hold a Chromebook in front of my face. I want to hold my students' joys and heartaches in my hands.

But I guess that's Your job, isn't it—virus or no virus? And Lord, You can teach them more at home in this sudden season than we could ever teach them in a normal school year. I think I needed that reminder. It's not about what I think they need, kind Father, but what You know they need.

Thank You, Lord, for providing for us, even in the middle of what we label loss. You've given us sweet, solid relationships with our students that will weather this storm, even when the waves block our view. And speaking of connection, You've given us the gift of technology—the ability to lecture and discuss and encourage from the safety of home. You've blessed us with supportive parents who are willing to partner with us in new ways during this season.

Father, although the force of this change stings, we affirm that You are still in control, that You are still good.

So, so good.

Teaching young students online is hard.

My uncle Elwood in Virginia, who has taught for nearly forty years, was also thrust into a new era of teaching. When I emailed him for advice, he simply said, "We figure these things out as we go."

That's one reason it was so hard. We—along with our city, state, and country—had to figure things out as we plodded along. If we tried one thing and it didn't work well, was there actually a better way, or was it simply something we had to deal with? And how do you do things well when so much is out of your control? There's not much we could do about crying babies in phonics class, lost math worksheets or scissors, weak internet connections, and cranky computers.

Our four-point vision statement at LARCS constantly reminded us of our goal for academic excellence. And constantly those words mocked us as we struggled to pull together screen-worthy classes that moved us beyond virtual babysitters to academic stimulators.

Miss Cindy wrestled with some of the biggest challenges as she taught first- and second-grade phonics and math. Even with small classes, it's tricky to teach young ones remotely. Over and over, however, Jesus reflected Himself in her patience.

Many weeks into online teaching, I stumbled onto an article that identified so well what I and thousands of others were facing: Zoom fatigue. Staring at screens, even screens full of faces you love, is exhausting. As relational beings, we rely on nonverbal communication to complement conversation. While video calls provide some of that, our minds strain to absorb it all while our eyes glaze over from the glare of the screen. We also, however unconsciously, strive harder to adequately communicate our thoughts to the other tiny tiles on the screen. Days with two classes in the morning and a Zoom teacher meeting in the afternoon proved more exhausting than I could initially understand. Even now, it's difficult to reconcile those short yet draining days with the long regular school days not many weeks before.

Teaching to blurry squares on the screen—sometimes only a shoulder or a forehead—was disheartening. When you can't understand each other, when papers fall out of binders, when students tussle on the mattress, or when the phone dies mid-class, engagement feels impossible. We eventually established helpful routines and incentives, but there were also things we simply had to let go.

But there were reasons to rejoice amid the unique challenges. Often our students' faith would bolster our own when we needed an infusion. Every day, the first and second graders could be heard praying for God to "please stop the coronavirus." They faithfully prayed for their teachers and that we could all be together soon.

We also enjoyed the unexpected evidence of solid relationships with our students and their parents. Had COVID swept in a year earlier, our ability to weather online learning could have been a different story. Our students' love and trust, coupled with their parents' support, were clear testimony of God's goodness and helped to ease the frustration of school on a screen.

And we smiled, too, at the sparks of humor during online classes, which I chronicled in my Fingerprint Files.

March 27

> Right now, nothing feels right or normal, so I relished the small comfort of these oh-so-normal words from Jonathan during the Duo call yesterday: "I can't find my pencil!" Some things never change.

March 30

> "Can I tell you something?" Kevin's face popped onto the screen just as I was ready to end the call. He told me he had memorized the first five verses of James 3, and then proudly recited it for Mr. Brendon and me.

Oh, that boy is hiding God's Word in his heart because he wants to. Thank You, Jesus.

May 20

Yesterday I told my class at the beginning of English Language Arts that we would begin with prayer.

"Miss Jess?" one seventh grader suddenly and uncharacteristically asked. "Can I pray tomorrow?"

So, this morning he was ready to pray when I asked him to. His prayer was short but full. He prayed God would "protect our hearts and minds." He also prayed for me as I taught. His words did my heart so much good.

God, we want to embrace each day as another opportunity to watch what You're going to do. Thank You for these glimpses into what You're doing in our students' hearts.

Online school ushered in new opportunities for family discipleship. School and home were no longer two distinct entities. School life became part of home life, which offered fresh ways to walk alongside our students' moms. These were challenging months for these women. Some were out of work and felt trapped at home, and others needed to work and feared exposure to the virus. Our biweekly homework drop-offs provided a few minutes of connection with these strong moms. Whether that meant giving a listening ear, praying for strength, or simply reorganizing student homework bins, we were given the gift of journeying with these beautiful women in practical ways.

While our vision of academic excellence stretched thin, the vision for family discipleship only swelled. Parents and staff alike discovered new commonalities as we each wrestled through the fears and complications of COVID. We were all in it together, held by the same God of grace.

Although there have been aches in this unexpected season, the throbs dull in comparison to what much of the world has experienced. While we missed face-to-face relationships, we still had a community. Even though our church didn't gather for ten Sundays, we still fellowshipped over Zoom and sought to creatively care for each other throughout the weeks. It hurts to think about how many people in this city had no one to knock on their door, bring them a gallon of milk, or share a kind word.

Our church community has been burdened for all the children affected by the rude shove of COVID. For many children, school was the only stable and safe place in their lives. It's a troubling thought that the Safer-at-Home orders and school shutdown may have spared physical health for a few at the cost of the emotional, spiritual, and social health of many at-risk children and teens in this city.

The school year wound down for us on June 11. That last week, we split into two groups for COVID-style field trips, relishing a taste of togetherness we all missed. After much discussion, we hosted a brief outdoor year-end ceremony for those who could attend, honoring our students for finishing their grades and bidding farewell to Miss Ruthann and Miss Cindy as teachers. All of us—students, parents, and teachers—were relieved to close the schoolbooks for the year as we anticipated a fresh school year beginning on August 18.

July 17

The first words of the message on the teacher group chat this afternoon didn't look promising. "I don't even know what to say," Benji wrote. "We need to pray lots and process this together. It's now illegal to do in-person schools in LA County. . . . "

As I skimmed over the lengthy article outlining Governor Newsom's order for all school campuses to close until COVID numbers came down, my mind and heart struggled to absorb the news. Schools were instructed to teach virtually until further notice, after which they may open campuses provided thirteen pages of guidelines are enforced.

This news means more than finding a better online teaching platform, more creative teaching techniques, and the ability to settle sibling squabbles virtually. It means journeying into a new phase of discipleship as we navigate these next months with our students and their parents. If our vision statement focused on mere academ-

> ics, this news would be crumpling. But family
> discipleship is at the top of the vision, and
> who but God would bring us into our students'
> homes in such a creative way?

This news harshly reminded us that the coronavirus is not yet just a few paragraphs of facts with neatly justified margins in a history book.

It's not yet a season we can glance back at and sigh, "Remember?" Rather, we're still peering around and asking, "Now what?"

The "now what?" plan for God's little school in Los Angeles is to homeschool in three different locations. Mr. Brendon will teach two students at school. I will teach four siblings in an extra room our pastor's family has graciously opened for our use. Miss Gwen will teach some mornings with me and other mornings with Maria as she homeschools her children.

It's not what we had planned, but we have confidence God is still working. Perhaps sometime soon LA County will accept waivers for schools. Perhaps the upcoming elections will shift the educational outlook in this city. Or perhaps God has simply called us to faithfully teach and disciple our students as He continues to teach us to trust and wait on Him.

This news also invites us to press into the challenges the Lord gives us in this season. Challenges as gifts? When glimpsed with hopeful eyes, eyes tilted toward the giver of all good gifts, challenges transform into gifts we were not creative enough to ask for. They flow into opportunities to watch God's grace spill into the daily and chances to gaze at the One who sustains when our humanity cries for change. And when we let God meet us in the challenges, in the brokenness of our understanding, and in the joy of dwelling in His will, there's no telling what He will do.

And They Did Eat

Shannon Hostetler

And, lo, the days of quarantine were upon them all,
and the tribe of Eric, son of Dan, did reside at home,
day after day after day upon day,
until the day turned into night, and night into morning,
with no knowledge of what day may be tomorrow,
neither could they tell what day was this very hour,
from the rising of the sun to the setting thereof.

And, behold, while they remained in the house,
they did roam about, searching for things to devour,
and the sound of munching and crunching
did fill the ears of all that were in the house.

And the mother of the tribe did weep and wail in lament,
saying unto herself and to all within hearing,
"How is it that the consumption of food is so great among us?
Shall I go out and sell all that we have to buy bread?
Whatever has overcome your stomachs
that you believe starvation to be nigh?"

And they answered her not, for they did not hear,
neither did they observe,
for the sound of their chewing was deafening.

And so it was, that day after day the mother of the tribe
did lean over the fire, cooking for the children of her youth.
And the consumption of the food thereof was great.

There were meats to be grilled, potatoes to be mashed,
squawking chickens to be plucked and cooked,
hamburgers to be prepared, while pasta and sauces simmered.
Cookies and pies, bread, bars, and cakes,
more cookies, along with fruit and veggies galore.
There were fried pancakes and eggs, sausage and bacon,
bowls of cereal, with bagels and muffins for all.
Great dishes of lasagna, heaping piles of chipotle,
pizza and steaks and roast beef with gravy,
along with all the leeks and garlic of Egypt.

Behold, they fared sumptuously every day,
and they did all eat but were not filled.

And turning, the mother wiped the sweat from her brow,
yet her eyes beheld not the fruits of her labor,
but only the crumbs that remained,
being licked up by the dog.

Disbelief and despair marked her face,
and upon seeing her look, her son wailed also:
"Mother, whence hath the food departed?
I find nothing at all to eat! Behold, I perish!"

And sitting down, she did put her head in her hands
and sighed greatly, saying,
"My son, I too am begging for an answer to thy question.
Who is the ravenous among us devouring it all?
For, lo, all my work has disappeared, eaten by people
roaming to and fro, looking for what they might devour.
What is this that has come upon us?"

And her cooking spirit did wither and fail,
and she rose from her chair with a heave and a sigh,
proclaiming to all within hearing, that
she was weary and worn and in need of much rest.
For never in all of her days had she beheld such a thing,
that the staying home of the tribe
had turned them into ravening wolves,
scavenging for food to be devoured before the night.

And with the voice of a trumpet, she did declare
them to be filled, fat, and full, and no food was to be eaten
until the serving of the next square meal.

And a great cry arose, but she did drown them out, saying,
"Get out thy books. Homeschool has begun!"

COVID-19 Adventure: Chapter One

Crystal Steinhauer

LIFE AS WE KNEW it changed—possibly forever—in the middle of March when the Belizean government announced that the borders, airports, and schools would shut down at the end of the week. Our imaginations ran wild. How deadly would this disease be? Certainly we wouldn't close church—that had never happened before. But I had always wanted to homeschool, so the prospect was exciting. My husband teaches at a mission school, and his salary comes from church offerings. If people couldn't go to church and give, would his salary end?

Talk of the virus dominated every conversation. The reaction of many in our village was fear. Many of the food-stand operators, street vendors, and taxi drivers immediately put their businesses on hold. Villagers even tried to stone a taxi driver who had driven customers to the Guatemalan border. No one he was in contact with had COVID-19, but if the borders were being closed, borders must be dangerous things.

I took some friends to town to stock up on groceries before lockdown. Along the way a woman stood beside her van holding a gas can, so we picked her up. Our lives were being disrupted; what did a little detour matter? In that moment I knew the virus would bring some positive effects that would help us to realize what was truly important.

Belize locked down on March 20, before the country had any cases. With the border closed, I worried about something happening to our families. What if one of our loved ones would die? Would we be able to attend the funeral?

The coronavirus felt like a blizzard—potentially dangerous, but kind of exciting. I bought prizes as incentives for our homeschool, and we set up a classroom on our porch. I enjoyed teaching and had always wanted to do more Bible memory with my children, so our school had an enthusiastic beginning.

We made brownies for a bedtime snack, grilled and ate outside more, played tree base in the yard, painted coconuts for a homemade bocce-ball game, and picked out new songs to learn as a family. Extensive news coverage of the growing number of cases in the United States seemed far away.

On March 31, Belize announced its first case—a woman who had flown back into the country from Los Angeles the week before. The government announced a State of Emergency, and began extensive mapping to find out who had been in contact with this woman. The authorities publicly scolded her for not self-quarantining as she was supposed to upon her return to Belize. I can only imagine the threats she must have received from the community.

A flurry of rumors followed the announcement of the State of Emergency. Some of my neighbors heard that all stores, even grocery stores, were going to close. Buses stopped running, except to carry employees to work, so my neighbors begged me to take them to town to stock up before everything closed. The first stores we passed required masks, and most stores were limiting the number of people allowed inside. Only one person per family—no children—was allowed in the stores. At some stores lines of people waited to get in.

The State of Emergency meant no one could go out on the street without an essential purpose. The police threatened people with a $5,000 fine and up to two years in prison if anyone violated the rules. Quite a few people were arrested in the cities for breaking curfew, but I never heard that those extreme consequences were actually imposed. The police asked one of our church men for some six-foot-long sticks to use to check for proper social distancing. Later we heard that their use had been expanded to whacking violators.

I began to shrivel under the new State of Emergency. My morning walks were now illegal. Our church did not have its own call-in service, so I felt increasingly isolated from our church people. I hated seeing the schoolroom doors barred. In some ways, my life hadn't changed much. We don't usually have a full social calendar, but not being able to go anywhere made me want to go *somewhere* in the worst way.

The case count in Belize slowly rose. When I went for groceries the next week, the police were stopping vehicles and asking drivers what their business was. If the police deemed it nonessential, they would ask the driver to turn around. I found it invasive and suffocating.

I struggled with feeling listless, unfocused, and depressed. I read in the news that Belize had its first coronavirus death. The wife of the deceased complained that the nurses had refused to care for her husband when they discovered he had COVID. Nurses complained that they were scared because they didn't have adequate personal protective equipment. I heard about ladies in the Unites States and Canada sewing masks and gowns for hospitals. I thought maybe that would give me some purpose, so I contacted my pediatrician, who gave me the number for the medical chief of staff at Northern Regional Hospital in Orange Walk.

I never got the call made, because the next day our plans flew out the window. The embassy announced that United Airlines was chartering a repatriation flight for US citizens in Belize. If we wanted to travel to the States within the next several months, this was our chance. We encouraged Geneva, the schoolteacher who lived with us, to take advantage of it. But the more we thought about it and talked to our families and church people, the more we felt that we should go as well.

After I bought the tickets, I walked around in a daze. How could we leave our Belize home? How could we leave the country we love at its most vulnerable moment? What if the disease would explode here? What if some of our church people would get sick or die?

Getting ready to leave for several months is so much more than packing suitcases. There were a million little things to do, such as collecting my baking sheets from neighbors who had borrowed them, making sure neighbors who were storing chicken in our freezer got it out, finding someone to stay overnight in the house while we were gone, labeling the dozens of keys so whoever stayed could figure them out, finding someone to care for our potted plants, and on and on.

I broke quarantine to take our excess groceries to a few neighbors; some of them were already in near-desperate condition because they had no work. One family had applied for the promised government aid, but so far hadn't heard anything. They were rationing their food, mostly ramen noodles. (Apparently they didn't know about the stockpiles of staples in each village that were meant for needy families.)

We were able to stop at most of the church people's homes to say goodbye in person, which helped bring closure. One of my regrets is that I never made it to Nevin and Wanda Yoder's home. Two months after we left, the cancer that had been slowly growing in her body wrapped its cold fingers around her and began to squeeze out the life. Her lungs started filling with fluid, and a medevac flight carried her back to the States, where she died at her son's home twelve days later. I never got to say goodbye.

When we booked our tickets, we pictured a normal flight, but in the days leading up to our trip, we realized this was going to be anything but normal. We filled out multiple forms for both the US embassy and the Belize government, and we occasionally received updates from both with more details about flight requirements.

Tuesday, two days before we were to leave, the Belize government notified us that since no private vehicles were allowed to drive to the airport, Tropic Air would fly us from the small airstrip in Orange Walk to the international airport. When we got the bill, it seemed as though the government wanted to profit from our flight—US$1,900 to fly our family the fifteen-minute hop. We reached out to the embassy, and they said they would do their best to make other travel arrangements.

We had a five o'clock deadline to pay for the Tropic Air tickets. Throughout the day we went back and forth with the embassy staff, who were trying to secure permission for us to go another way. Twenty minutes before the deadline, I sent a desperate message to our families, asking them to pray. Five minutes later, we got an email from the Belize government letting us know they would provide bus transportation for us from Orange Walk to the airport for BZ$50 (US$25) a person. That was more like it! My neighbors gawked as I ran out the door waving my phone and shouting, "THANK YOU, JESUS!"

On Thursday, April 16, we said goodbye to our Belize home. One of the men from church took us to the meeting place in town where we joined the others from Orange Walk district who were flying out. A bus carried us to the airport.

The airport was a six-foot-spaced-apart maze of waiting for this document and that paper. When we finally had our passports updated and forms filled out, we had been standing in lines for three hours, and my nerves were already frazzled.

When we boarded the plane, I discovered that we had not been assigned seats together, even though I had paid extra for the privilege, so we had to ask people to move so our younger children could be near us.

I had taken my mask off to relax a minute; then my seatmate arrived. She scowled at me. "Don't you have a mask?" So back on went the mask. She was an irritable seatmate, and I developed a serious headache, which was compounded by my baby not sleeping during the flight.

We had heard the airports were nearly empty. It was almost eerie to land in Houston and find we were the only international flight going through immigration. We were through in a few minutes, and if I had blinked, I would have missed customs, which consisted of one woman asking if anyone had plants or seeds and then waving us through.

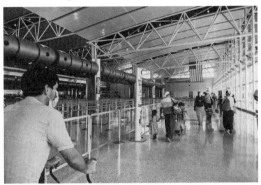

Empty Immigration in Houston

The airport had a forlorn atmosphere, with few travelers and many of the stores and restaurants closed. I had worried about the children picking up germs in the airport, but there were few people and plenty of cleaning staff wiping surfaces.

We got a hotel for the night, where we ordered takeout from Pizza Hut and coffees from Burger King, slept in luxuriously large beds, and used as much water as we wished without worrying about our cistern running dry. I got up before everyone else and enjoyed the most delicious culture shock by taking a walk down a landscaped street, occasionally crossing sides to avoid sprinklers.

From Houston we flew to Washington, DC, and then to Harrisburg, PA, only half an hour from my parents' home. The flight from Belize to Houston cost far more than normal, but we were able to get from Houston to Harrisburg for twenty dollars a person.

What a joy to see my parents drive up to the airport! We said goodbye to Geneva and headed to our lovely cabin in the woods, where we self-quarantined for two weeks. My family had outdone themselves by stocking the cabin with everything we needed for a comfortable stay.

Quarantine was not a hardship. We loved tramping through the woods, and everything was new and exciting. I often felt a little guilty as we sat by the crackling fire during the unusually cold April weather while our Belizean friends endured temperatures over one hundred degrees every day, extreme drought, and smog from forest fires.

Our biggest culture shock was the way Pennsylvanians were reacting to the virus. We had been carefully taking precautions—trying to stay home, wearing masks, using sanitizer. Many in our village were genuinely scared for their lives and couldn't imagine why we would travel to the States during this time when, according to what they had heard on the news, it sounded as if people were dropping dead like flies. Belizeans carefully followed government regulations, both because they were frightened and also because the police strictly enforced things such as curfew. It was a bit of a shock to discover that some Pennsylvanians thought the virus was a hoax, and most felt it was a media exaggeration. They seemed to pick and choose which regulations they followed.

So ends chapter one of our COVID-19 adventure. During lockdown, no one we knew died or even got sick. But since then, dozens of acquaintances have gotten sick. We also put in some time on the couch and learned what it's like to live without taste and smell. We are still unsure of when we will be able to return to Belize. We are all getting a little homesick, although being "stuck" in the States has been far from unpleasant. What will chapter two hold? I have no idea. Thankfully, God does.

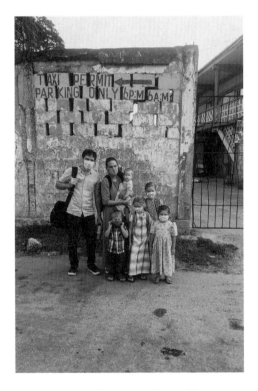

The Steinhauer Family in Belize

Open Hands

Stacey LaSee

AS I STOOD IN line to register at Sharon Mennonite Bible Institute, I picked up a Fourth Term schedule and leaned against the wall, scanning the events planned for the next six weeks. Anticipation welled inside me as I noted the opportunities: Missions Conference, church visitation, a choir program. It looked to be a full term, ending with a three-week choir tour that would take us out west.

Other students gathered around the office, examining syllabus papers or chatting about classes. *It's odd to think I'll actually know all these people by the end of six weeks. . . .* I had attended three terms at SMBI over the past few years, but the roster hanging on the wall assured me there would be more students this time than I had ever gone with before—seventy-two in all. I wondered how this term would be different from the previous ones.

"Stacey LaSee?" the secretary called. "You can register in Cliff's office now."

I stepped into the administrator's office to go over my class choices and other details. I knew the next weeks would fly by, but I was eager to get started.

I filed through the food line in the kitchen and then entered the dining room to find a seat. Halfway to one of the tables for eight, I suddenly remembered. *Oh, that's right. We're having a meeting over supper.* Turning around, I set my tray on one of the long tables on the other side of the room. Jenna came out of the kitchen and sat beside me. The two of us, along with three others, were on a committee to plan a children's skit to do on tour during the intermission of our choir programs.

The first three weeks of the term had gone by as scheduled, and I enjoyed the rhythm of my classes, choir, and homework. It was now Monday of the fourth week, and though the weekend had been good, I was glad to be back in the swing of things.

"So has anyone come up with any ideas?" Jonny asked, when we were all assembled.

We hashed over possibilities, and before long, we agreed on the "You are Special" story and a children's song to go with it. The potential excited me, but just then Cliff stood to make some announcements.

"I'm sure you've all heard about the coronavirus, right?" Cliff began with a wry grin. We all looked at each other with knowing glances. Of course, we knew about it, but it was just some random thing going on somewhere else. ""Well, it's now beginning to directly affect us," he said. "New policies are being put in place throughout the country to try to control the disease, and we have a responsibility to do what's required of us. Starting tonight, we are instating a no-visitor policy, and students are not to leave campus to go into town more than they have to."

I usually stayed around the school anyway, so this new restriction was not a big deal for me. Cliff was not finished, however. "Because we can't have visitors and must limit our interaction with the public, church visitation for this weekend and the choir program scheduled for next week have been canceled. As far as tour, we don't know if we can still go at this point, but with everything that keeps popping up, it looks highly unlikely. Are there any questions?"

Alex raised his hand. "The food committee was planning to make food for tour tonight. Should we still do that?"

"I would hold off on it for now," Cliff replied.

My thoughts were in turmoil. No longer was the coronavirus simply a world crisis. It had just gotten personal.

"I kind of like this no-visitor thing," I said to a friend as we stood in line for lunch. "Now that it's just us and we're all stuck here together, maybe we can get to know everybody better."

"Yeah, I guess," she reluctantly agreed, "but I was looking forward to having my sister come visit this weekend."

"Oh, I'm sorry," I said. I could see how disappointing that would be, but I was from the faraway state of Wisconsin, so I didn't have anyone coming to see me anyway.

Signs declaring "Closed to visitors (until further notice)" had been posted on the school doors, and life had gone on while I grappled with the disappointments of church visitation and our choir program being canceled. But the hardest adjustment was the thought of the tour being canceled too. It hadn't worked out for me to come for Fourth Term and the three-week tour last year, so I had transferred my application to this term. After planning on this for over a year, I struggled to leave it in God's hands.

I smiled, recalling the student-led prayer meeting the evening of Cliff's announcement, and the blessed time of sharing, singing, and praying we'd had. God had given me peace as I surrendered the tour to Him, and every day He was patiently teaching me the truth of Proverbs 16:9: "A man's heart deviseth his way: but the LORD directeth his steps."

Things had settled to a new normal, and trouble seemed far away as I sat in my early-morning class that Friday, taking notes while we discussed the temptations of Jesus. But as our teacher, Byron, stressed a certain point, he suddenly choked up. "This may be our last class together," he said, "and I want you all to remember this . . . ."

Our last class? I glanced at the other students, but no one else seemed to know what was happening, either. Byron continued with the teaching, but my mind was awhirl for the rest of the class period. *Whatever is going on will probably be announced at chapel directly after this,* I decided, and I was right.

"Last night, there were new developments," Cliff informed us. "The governor of Pennsylvania announced that all non-life-sustaining businesses are to be closed because of the coronavirus. It's uncertain how the school is considered in relation to that, but the SMBI board has checked with law enforcement about what we are to do. The trooper said he'll look into it and let us know by three o'clock this afternoon. Meet here in the chapel again at four o'clock, and by then we should know what the verdict will be."

I tried to absorb the shock. If we couldn't continue as we were, we would all have to leave within twenty-four hours and not be able to finish out the term! The thought of leaving classes unfinished and making such a quick departure looked overwhelming.

Somehow, I made it through my classes, and even did homework in between, although I wondered if it was necessary. Directly after fourth-period class, I joined the others assembling in the chapel to hear the verdict. The day had crawled by in a haze of uncertainty, and I was glad the suspense would soon be over.

The atmosphere was tense as the minutes ticked by. Finally, Cliff walked up to the podium and surveyed our serious expressions. "I feel like I'm at a press conference," he said dryly. "Well, I'm going to give you the answer and then explain the reasoning behind it." He paused. "We don't know."

I heaved a sigh of relief. The pressure in the room suddenly dropped as we realized we weren't being sent home the next day.

"The trooper called back and said we're in a gray area," Cliff explained, "but he doesn't have a definite answer for us. So, while the SMBI board will be on the watch for any new directives, we'll continue in our self-imposed isolation as we have been until further notice."

"So, we really don't know anything more now than we did before," a student commented to me when we were dismissed.

"True, but at least we can stay," I said, grateful that, while the future was still unsettled, the stress of the day had been defused.

Grabbing a book from my dorm room, I headed downstairs to do some assigned reading. I knew the final decision about choir tour would be made by this evening, so I went to check if anything new had been posted about it. The possibility of the term itself being cut short had overshadowed that issue for the time being, but I still felt a stab of disappointment as I read the new update on our situation: "While we continue to function under a significant degree of uncertainty, our current position is stable enough that it is possible to present some tentative schedules for the remainder of the term...." I wasn't surprised to see that the tour had been canceled, but now that the door was officially shut, the loss sank in.

"At least we can still do a live-streamed program next Wednesday," someone observed.

"And we get to record on Friday before leaving," I pointed out. "That's a blessing I didn't think we'd be able to have." I settled down to my homework, feeling as if that schedule was something I could live with. We could still do a program and record, too. Or, at least, that was the plan....

"How are you all doing on holding things with open hands?" Cliff asked as we lined up for supper the last Saturday of the term.

I cringed. Holding life with open hands had become a theme among us as we realized that every additional day we could stay was indeed a blessing from the Lord. But something in Cliff's tone indicated he had hard news to break to us. Sure enough, it was another jolting announcement.

"New restrictions have come up here in Pennsylvania with some more counties added to the stay-at-home order," Cliff informed us. "So, the board of SMBI has been discussing things. The result has been a significant change of course for us. Instead of ending with recording on Friday, we need to wrap up everything by Wednesday and send you all home on Thursday."

And we won't be able to record the songs we've practiced for weeks and put hours of work into?

Cliff went on. "The good news is that we still have approval to live-stream the choir program on Wednesday. We can be thankful for that opportunity."

I *was* glad for that, but struggled in dealing with yet another adjustment, another shattered hope. By this time, I should have been used to changing plans, but the loss hurt. It was another upheaval on the emotional roller coaster I'd been riding the past couple of weeks.

Entering the public lounge early the next morning, I joined a group of others who had decided to trade some extra sleep for the chance to go to a nearby lookout and watch the sunrise. After waiting for several stragglers, Wynn gave the go-ahead to start loading into vehicles for the ride over.

The lookout was one I'd been at twice during past terms at SMBI. The first time, I had gone with a group after dark to see the lights across the valley. The other time, a friend and I had gone in the afternoon to spend some time together. I knew what the view was like during the day and at night, but when I arrived this time, I saw nothing. No beautiful valley with mountains rising in the distance. No panorama of lights shining across the darkened landscape. Only fog. Dense, low-hanging clouds completely obscured the view, along with any possibility of seeing the sunrise. A fine mist was falling, and the air was cold.

Somehow, I'm not surprised, I mused. *It's just another thing that isn't going to turn out as planned.* But as I sat on one of the rocks and joined the others in singing, I sensed God was using this to show me something. Someone suggested singing "I Believe,"[5] one of our choir songs. I listened as Kiersten began with the solo, and then the sopranos joined her: "I believe in the sun, even when it's not shining."

With the backdrop, and what we'd been experiencing throughout term, it was a powerful moment as those words rang out. I joined the altos on the second verse: "I believe in love, even when I don't feel it."

Then Kiersten took up the ending solo, "I believe in God, even when God is silent."

As the closing notes faded away, I realized that in the same way the term had been so uncertain, my future also looked like the foggy abyss in front of me; I couldn't see what was ahead. Maybe I didn't understand what God was doing and struggled with laying down my own plans in exchange for His will, but through the disappointments and pain, I had a choice to make. Would I turn away from God in confusion, angry that He didn't come through for me, or would I let go and trust everything into His capable hands?

---

5   Anonymous, "I Believe."

As we headed back to SMBI, I was grateful we didn't see the sunrise. The experience of worshipping God in the fog and mist was something I never want to forget.

We stood on risers in the front of the gym. Almost surprisingly, the schedule for the last few days of term had held out, and we were about to begin the live-streamed choir program. Our audience, seated in one of the back corners, consisted only of staff and the students who weren't in choir. On the opposite side, Friedrich and Logan manned a table of cords and electronics, while two cameras on tripods faced us at different angles. I smiled, thinking what a unique experience this was.

Finally, it was time. Andrew, our choir director, introduced the program, and we began. Singing for a mostly unseen audience was strange, but we understood this would be our only chance to do this. We wanted God to be glorified in it.

During intermission, most of us headed into the dining room to wait during Cliff's devotional.

"On my way out, I checked to see how many people are watching," Lavern said, his eyes lit with excitement. "There are over a thousand!"

"Seriously?" I exclaimed. "God has given us the opportunity to reach more people with one program than we would have on tour!" I was awed at the glimpse of how far God's ways are above our own.

Just before we sang "I Believe" in the second half of our program, I raised my hand for the microphone and gave a testimony about our Sunday morning excursion to the lookout. "The fog, in a lot of ways, depicts our future, especially in these times where a lot of things have changed.... And so, I just want you to be able to take in the message of this song and realize that God's love reaches out to you even when it seems at times that He is silent."

I handed the microphone back, and as I waited for the director to begin the song, I pondered how the term had turned out to be a far cry from what I'd imagined. But with the upheaval of the coronavirus and the "classes" I'd gone through that I didn't sign up for, God had taught me valuable life lessons about faith, trust, and holding life with open hands.

A Homeschooling Thermometer

Mabel Reiff

IT WAS MARCH, and I was finally ready to tackle projects such as sewing and writing. I wanted to try some new recipes before picking summer's bounty had us scurrying from dawn to dusk. I wanted coffee-break moments without guilt.

It didn't happen. COVID-19 happened instead. It canceled school and stole my anticipated time.

The first week out of school was glorious. There were no lessons assigned for the children yet, and they delighted in the unexpected vacation. Here in Lancaster County, Pennsylvania, the sun shone as warmly as in May, and I couldn't take time for sewing or coffee. Instead, I made the most of my available help by planting peas and tilling the soil for seeding grass where we had taken down an old shed last fall. We were busy outdoors a lot, and I loved working with my children as if it were summer vacation.

Then another Monday brought the first set of lessons and the start of a rainy, chilly season. I had never considered homeschooling, but I wasn't too concerned, since I had enjoyed four terms of teaching before marriage. Now, even with three preschoolers—which included a toddler and a six-month-old—I thought I could do it. I pictured my scholars seated around the kitchen table, diligently finishing each lesson. But I soon learned that teaching school at school, and homeschooling children accustomed to a school setting, were not the same thing.

It started well enough. Three boys and a girl, each with a stack of books and a list of assignments, settled around the table after lunch. I helped them find the right lessons and went back to the dishes. Yes, it started well.

"Mom! He kicked me," first-grader Hannah shrieked, glaring at Javan.

The eighth grader glared back. "I just pushed her with my foot, because she keeps humming and it drives me crazy. Anyway, I don't know how to do this."

I sat down beside him and studied the math that had once been as familiar to me as the children sitting around my table. We wasted time paging back to find the lesson with the instructions. Meanwhile, two-year-old Josiah sat on the table, rearranging stacks of books.

"He's getting my stuff!" Hannah grabbed her books and put them on the bench beside her. Josiah started to cry.

"I don't know how to do this." Lucas shoved his fifth-grade math book under my nose. "We never had it." He scowled at five-year-old Caleb in the chair beside his. "I don't *like* when people sit so close to me."

"Wait your turn." I dug out a coloring book and crayons for Caleb, who then decided he didn't want to color. I found the page for Javan and showed him how to start. Schoolwork had never been his strong point, and I had expected he would need more help. But Lucas should remember…

"I have a question." Hannah pointed to a math problem. "What is this answer?"

I told her to wait while I gave Lucas a quick rundown of his work, which did match an earlier lesson. Josiah clung to my leg, begging to be picked up. I held him and looked at Hannah's book. "Six plus two?" I tried to be patient. This was Hannah, who had read at a second-grade level before she started school. Why didn't she know her math facts?

"Eight?" She cheerfully wrote the answer that I suspected she had known all along. I set Josiah on the bench beside Hannah so I could pick up Baby Marcus. I put him in the clip-on high-chair so he would feel included. Javan needed help again.

Josiah cried. Third-grader Jethro tapped his pencil. Hannah started to hum again. Marcus fussed.

"Be quiet!" Lucas jumped up and rummaged in Daddy's sock drawer for earplugs. He found a pair and jammed them into his ears. Then Jethro needed some. He stuck one into his ear, pulled out a blob of wax, and showed it to Lucas.

"Yuck!" Lucas yelled, watching in fascination as Jethro proceeded to smear it across the corner of his page.

Javan got up to look for another eraser. As he passed Hannah, he yanked her braid. I felt pressure building inside me. "Grab your eraser and get back here." I picked up Marcus and sat on the couch to feed him with Josiah nestled beside me. "Lucas and Jethro, get busy." My voice sounded sharp to my ears; I cringed and took a deep breath.

Cold, rainy days followed. Some were better than others, but with the children cooped up inside so much, I struggled to keep a lid on my frustration. Little puffs of steam escaped here and there. I felt guilty when I heard how others were enjoying this time together at home as a family, while I struggled to keep ours from irritating one other. I even felt guilty for rejoicing that my carpenter son wasn't totally laid off, and that my second son was another farmer's right-hand man. I didn't need anyone else at home right now, especially since Daddy was still at his winter job. I desperately wanted time to clean or cook without having to keep the peace, without having to decide which were real needs of children who became attention deprived as soon as I helped a sibling. In truth, I resented the loss of time for myself.

"If you'd keep busy, you'd be done," I scolded Lucas, who sat staring at his open math book and an almost-blank notebook page at four o'clock one afternoon. It was the only lesson he had worked on all day. When he burst into tears, I felt a stab of remorse. For the first time, I realized I was not the only one struggling to adjust to this change in our schedule.

One day in a precious moment of silence, I dialed the number for the ten-minute inspirational message my mother-in-law had told me about. The speaker started with, "Are you a thermometer or a thermostat?" What? He didn't allow me to wonder long before he explained.

"A thermometer reflects the temperature of a room. A thermostat controls the temperature."

Oh. I pictured myself scolding and nagging and inwardly fuming while the red line of mercury climbed dangerously close to the top. No doubt about it; I had reacted to my circumstances instead of being in charge of my children as a Christian mother should be. I was turning into a human thermometer because of my selfish longing to do my own thing.

That night as I fed Marcus, I pondered the situation in a way that only the night hours allow one to do. I pictured each of my school-age children destined for a life of counselor appointments. Each of them would start with, "You see, all my problems began during the COVID-19 pandemic when my mom tried to homeschool us..."

I felt horrible. I prayed. I planned. The next morning I got up with fresh determination. I set goals and separated my children. "You go into the playroom, you go to the living room, and you two sit at opposite ends of the table." Instead of trying to juggle toddlers and lessons, I assigned the older children to babysit by turns. Consequences awaited anyone who distracted any person doing lessons, and I made sure those consequences were less than desirable.

That was the turning point. We still had rough edges that irritated each other, but the good days outnumbered the bad. We started to laugh at the new words we were learning, and we tried to use them in everyday conversations: *social distancing*, *pandemic*, *mandatory*, and *lockdown*.

When wearing masks in public became mandatory, we picked out fabric from the scrap box. I found space in an afternoon to sew one for each of us, except for Baby Marcus. We tried them on and wondered if we would get used to the feeling of not being able to breathe with all that warm air confined in front of our faces, steaming up our glasses.

We caught up on the cleaning and the garden weeds. Most of all, we started to enjoy each other again.

We ended the school term with the usual sighs of relief, which had nothing to do with schooling at home. Although I secretly prayed that schools would reopen in the fall, my third grader confided that he hoped we would continue to homeschool.

Toilet-paper shortages, stifling masks, and unexpected home-schooling shouldn't matter. Even a confining pandemic can't change our attitudes and family relationships unless we allow it to. If we need to homeschool again, by God's grace we'll manage—as long as Mom doesn't turn into a thermometer.

House Church

Sarah J. Martin

"TIME FOR CHURCH," called the patriarch. The tiny congregation gathered on a circle of chairs at one end of the dining room. The matriarch noted the sock feet of everyone save the youth girl beside her, who was sockless in high heels.

The young members of the group squirmed, then settled down. The patriarch turned to the youth boy. "Do you have a song picked out?"

"Yup. Number 481. I found four songs about Psalm 91, and this is the only one we know." He looked at his sister across from him. "You have your phone with the pitch-pipe app?"

She didn't. So they all waited while the intermediate boy darted up the stairs, looking for his father's pitch pipe. Meanwhile, the youth downloaded one on his phone. It was just as well, for the physical one had disappeared.

When the intermediate boy returned, the service began. "There is a safe and secret place, / Beneath the wings divine. ..." Mature and childish voices rose in harmony, singing the timeless hymn. "O child of God, O glory's heir, / How rich a lot is thine!"[6]

The baby's sippy cup fell and rolled across the "auditorium." The youth boy curled his toes around the handle and tossed it to the mother, who missed. The cup clattered distractingly before the mother snatched it up.

"For a devotional, let's turn to Psalm 91," said the patriarch. "We'll take turns reading the verses. You may start," he told the primary-age boy.

"'He that dwelleth in the secret place of the most High shall abide under the shadow of the Almighty.'" Around the circle they read, youthful voices and deep ones making the words come alive.

When it was the mother's turn to read, she paused. Did she need to swallow emotions? "'Nor for the pestilence that walketh in darkness; nor for the destruction that wasteth at noonday,'" she read, hoping the tremor in her voice was imperceptible. Such a relevant psalm. She thought of the dear souls gathered around her, and of the sinister virus that stalked the world in those days.

But that promise: "Thou shalt not be afraid. . . ." She took a deep breath.

"'With long life will I satisfy him, and shew him my salvation.'" The words of the last verse hung in the air. The congregation pondered.

"So," said the patriarch, "if one of us gets the coronavirus, does that mean Psalm 91 isn't true?"

---

6   Henry F. Lyte, "There Is a Safe and Secret Place."

The answer was unanimous: "No."

"If one of us dies from it, is Psalm 91 still true?"

Again, no hesitation: "Yes."

The youth boy spoke up. "It doesn't say we won't get sick; it just says we won't be afraid." True. So true.

After a prayer, the Sunday school class clattered down the stairs to the rec room, with the youth girl in charge. The senior members and the youth boy moved to the living room adjacent to the makeshift sanctuary to study the instruction lesson about prayer and fasting.

Half an hour elapsed. The singing from downstairs was interspersed with giggles and off-key notes, the Sunday school class obviously over. The patriarch had considered doing a second instruction lesson, but decided to call the Sunday school class back to the auditorium after the matriarch said, "It sounds as if the teacher is just putting in time down there."

While the juniors and primaries returned, the patriarch meandered down the hall, looking at his phone. The youth boy looked at his, too, and announced news from other house churches.

"We don't generally catch up on our phones during a church service," whispered the matriarch. She and the patriarch shared sheepish looks, and the phones disappeared.

Shuffling and quiet arguments ensued as the tiny congregation assembled once more, but finally all the members were satisfied with the general decision to remain in the chairs they had previously occupied.

The songs ministered to their hearts again as they sang "I Know the Lord Will Make a Way for Me" and "Great Is Thy Faithfulness." The preschool girl sang an octave above the other sopranos, her earnest face the picture of worship. The toddler, despite repeated untwisting by the matriarch, sat backward on his twirling stool and stuck gum on the hutch doors. When he threatened to cause a disaster by probing the dishes, she took him onto her lap.

After the songs, the tribe was dismissed to various activities. Soon they would return to eat the steak and potatoes that were sending delicious aromas through the house. But for now, a moment of peace. The matriarch sat down to write about the church service.

"I Want the Lord to Have His Way with Me,"[7] they had sung. It was not their choice to have church this way, but they found comfort in the inspiration and blessing God had given them.

And why not? Jesus said, "For where two or three are gathered...." He is worthy of worship even in these strange days, and perhaps more now than ever before.

---

7   Anonymous, "I Know the Lord Will Make a Way."

Social Distancing and Compassion

Elfreda R. Showalter

"IF YOU ARE PAYING with cash, PLEASE don't lick your fingers," read the bold signs in the entryway and checkout line at a local store.

In the town of Farmington, New Mexico, grocery shopping during COVID-19's first weeks was a maze. The confusion sidetracked my thoughts from my list. Shopping with people who were masked and gloved and trying to stay six feet apart gave me a weird feeling.

Finally, I had gathered what I needed. I made my way to the checkout. Oh, those social-distancing lines! I looked down at the marks on the floor and stopped with the front of my cart six feet behind the shopper ahead of me. "Good!" I congratulated myself. "I followed that rule."

My satisfied feeling was short-lived. The shopper in front took one look at me and promptly headed my way. *Am I supposed to back up?* The masked face came toward me until her toes crossed the social-distancing line into my space. She put her gloved hands on my cart, leaned toward me over my groceries, and whispered through her bandana-style mask, "You have my condolences in relation to Sasha Krause's death."

I found my voice after my brain jerked out of its initial distress. I thanked her profusely and added, "We still miss her very much!"

She returned to the checkout and paid for the groceries the clerk had rung up in her absence. Her heart was warm even if her mask made her look like a kidnapper.

Amazing! I thought. My mind had been occupied with finding my groceries, but this lady was thinking beyond herself. She saw me and knew that the only Mennonites in the surrounding towns were from the church where the Sunday school teacher had been kidnapped eight weeks earlier. My heart warmed to know the community still cared deeply about what had happened.

Over the loudspeaker came the reminder, "We are in this together." Though it was said in reference to COVID-19, I thought of how brokenhearted the community was about Sasha Krause's disappearance. Together, we had waited five weeks to learn what had become of her. Together, we had mourned the heart-wrenching discoveries. People who did not personally know Sasha shed many tears.

Walmart's one-way aisles demand a lot of extra walking. If a product is within sight—maybe only a yard away—but the red sign on the floor says "Do Not Enter," I must walk the length of the next aisle, turn the corner, enter the green zone, and walk down that aisle to get what I need. On one of these excursions, someone called, "I want to talk to you!" A little white-haired lady pulling her cart against the designated flow of traffic motioned for me to stop. She won my heart right away; she looked too old to be shopping alone.

The pink-suited grandma sidled up to me to murmur through her mask about Sasha Krause—after all, it isn't proper to stand six feet apart to discuss a dear friend who had been kidnapped and murdered. She squeezed my elbow and patted my arm at fitting moments in her inquiry about how we members of the Farmington church were coping with our loss.

I couldn't back farther away because I was against a shelf and my cart. Other shoppers gave us you've-got-to-be-crazy looks as they passed by with purpose. The voice over the loudspeaker reminded shoppers from time to time, "All loitering inside and outside the store is strictly forbidden."

"I wanted to come to that memorial service your church had, but I didn't make it," she lamented. "I want to hug you," she added. And hug she did. The moment we embraced, she remembered the COVID-19 regulations. "Oh, I'm so sorry." She moved to the proper six-foot distance. "I remember to wear my mask, but I'm always forgetting to stay back from people. I'm perfectly fine in my health—as far as I know."

And with a chuckle and a wave, she hurried on her way, heading in the wrong direction down the aisle.

A few minutes later, I came within twenty feet of her again. She waved from afar and called, "I'll remember to stay six feet away from you this time." She chuckled, and I went home smiling. I frowned the next day when I needed the flour I had missed while talking to her. But my smile returned when I realized the encounter was worth an extra trip. I smiled even more a few weeks later when I learned I had escaped the virus, even though a stranger had hugged me in the grocery store.

COVID-19 Wedding

Barbie Stoltzfus

WHEN OUR OLDEST daughter, Susan, became engaged, I was thrilled, but then reality set in. Lord willing, a wedding follows an engagement. For members of the Lancaster County Amish, planning a wedding is not for the faint of heart. Typically, the first guest arrives at six thirty in the morning, and the last one leaves around nine o'clock at night. Two full-course meals are served to more than four hundred guests, besides refreshments in the afternoon. All this is planned by the bride's mother, who in this case was me—disorganized, scatterbrained, baby-of-the-family me.

Traditions help with the planning and organizing of a wedding. Without fail, a wedding is planned for a Tuesday or Thursday, from November through March. For the noon meal, chicken filling, cooked celery, coleslaw, and mashed potatoes are served. Since there are close to thirty-six thousand Amish in Lancaster County, once or twice someone might have broken the tradition and served something else. Or maybe someone invited only two hundred people. For years, I had wished to meet them—if such folks existed—to ask them if they thought it was worth the hassle of breaking the tradition. I secretly thought there must be an easier way to get married than to endure so much work and fuss. And I detested cooked celery.

"Do we need to be traditional?" my daughter asked. "Couldn't we have a small wedding that would seem like a backyard barbecue? But probably it's easier to be traditional than have the people fuss," she conceded.

Always before in my life, I could consult my older sisters about any major life changes or decisions. They were two jumps ahead, which had its advantages. They went to school first, and by the time I came along, they were experts at math and happy to assist me. They were experienced with teenage-girl drama and boyfriend woes before my turn came. Potty training, bed-wetting, and teenage attitudes had been their lot before it was mine, and I considered their advice the knowledge of experts.

But they were not experienced in the world of weddings. Our daughter was the first niece on both sides of the family to get married.

After her engagement, people occasionally asked if I was giggling to myself that I was about to do something my sisters had never done.

"No," I replied. "I'll wait till after the fact." What if it would be chaos? But it was a good opportunity to show my siblings that disorganized babies like me could change.

I had been to weddings that were organized and to weddings that were quite the opposite. I wanted ours to be the former. It was time to change my ways and to grow up. How hard could it be to teach myself to be more focused and organized? I borrowed four books and notes from ladies whose daughters had recently married. For hours I studied them and compared the notes scribbled in them.

I dug out a bright-red notebook from the attic and boldly printed "Wedding Planner" on the front with a Sharpie. Compiling my finds from the borrowed ones, I started my own with lists and notes that applied to my daughter's wedding.

I dreamed *wedding* in my sleep. I became absentminded in all conversations that didn't contain the word *wedding*.

"The wedding is still five months away," my husband pointed out one evening as I halfheartedly joined in the supper-table conversation. "You will be burned out before the time arrives."

I grinned to myself. I would show him.

"I wish we had twelve daughters," I told him. "Planning a wedding is so fun."

He snorted. "We'll discuss this again once the wedding is over. Then we'll see if you're still wishing for twelve daughters and twelve weddings."

We were invited to a host of fall weddings, and I attended with anticipation. I put a paper and pen in my pocket, and I sneaked into corners to jot down things I did or didn't like.

I talked with other mothers who were also having spring weddings, and I felt I was right on schedule. This wasn't hard.

I went shopping for wedding products, and as I carried them into the house, I twisted my ankle. It hurt, so I took time out to put ice on it and elevate it. The next morning I had only minimal discomfort, which I ignored. Twenty-four hours later, I could not walk on it. A week later, as I looked at the schedule I had mapped out for the next month, I took a deep breath and told myself to stay calm. I was four days behind schedule.

My sisters—the ones I wanted to impress—came and cleaned house. Several kind friends joined them. I was back on schedule.

After three days of being back to work full force, I noticed a slight sore throat and a dry cough. I was so tired by evening that I collapsed into bed, wondering what I enjoyed about wedding planning.

The next morning I had a fever. I headed for the couch and spent a week there. I was too sick to care about keeping schedules and impressing sisters, or proving a point to my husband.

The flu ran its course, and wedding planning resumed. I was a week behind schedule. My sisters bailed me out a second time.

At the supper table one evening in late February, my husband and oldest son discussed a strange sickness occurring in China. I thought about my doughnut platters—doughnuts with icing in spring colors—with chocolate Easter eggs wrapped in foil.... People were dying from this strange disease; I felt sorry for the Chinese.... My daughter wanted navy tablecloths with gold runners.... I needed to call the cook-trailer rental company to make sure that the dishes were white. Several of the older cook trailers had ancient green dishes called Melmac. These dishes had given me the willies ever since I was a little girl.

My men discussed the Chinese illness several times over the next week. I didn't pay much attention. China was an ocean away. When the first case came into the United States, followed in rapid succession by many more, I started paying more attention. It's hard to ignore a topic if you sit through a whole dinner-table conversation where nothing else is discussed. I even remembered the name of the illness—COVID-19. It sounded nasty. But since the only people affected by it were in big cities, it still seemed worlds away.

My days were consumed by cleaning, food prep, and outdoor work as we forged ahead to the final countdown.

Ten days before the wedding, schools were closed statewide in hopes of slowing down the epidemic that was spiraling out of control. There were still no cases in Lancaster County, so I wasn't alarmed that it would affect us in a major way. Except there was no school. I love my energetic seven-year-old, with his imagination and endless pranks. But I love him just as much when he's in school.

The day after the schools shut down, restaurants closed across the state. Nonessential businesses were next. My husband and I became alarmed when he heard at work that limiting crowds to a small size, though not mandatory, was strongly encouraged.

We attended a wedding the day after nonessential businesses had shut down, and multiple people wondered what we were going to do about our daughter's wedding. "We'll pray for you," they assured us, and I felt their love and concern. It was realistic to believe that the large wedding might not happen anytime soon.

I slept fitfully, if at all.

The wedding had been planned for Tuesday, March 24, 2020.

After two days of stressing, getting opinions from government officials and, finally, the green light to go ahead, we decided at precisely 2:30 p.m. on Wednesday, March 18, to have the wedding on Friday, March 20, with two hundred fewer guests.

The food list, which had taken me hours to prepare, was altered in fifteen minutes. Port-a-pots and horse tents had to be canceled for the original date and reordered. Wonder of wonders, I wasn't able to get celery in time to prepare cooked celery. I chose peas and carrots instead. As we prepared the food, I heard two family members moan that they couldn't imagine eating chicken filling without cooked celery. I was jealous that this was their biggest problem of the day.

The cook trailer and wedding tent were canceled for good. We decided to have the wedding out back in our shop. Our dirty, cobwebby shop. Family and friends descended on our property to clean and cook, snatching my careful plans and precious schedule from my hands.

The bride-to-be, recovering from a nasty flu, looked as impressed as I felt.

In frustration I cried out to God. "How is this fair? This should be a happy time for all of us, and my daughter needed next week to recover from the flu before her wedding. Now You are allowing this."

The day before the wedding, I alternated between wanting to cry and laughing long and loud.

The morning of the wedding, I—the bride's mother, who was expected to be calm and serene with a happy smile on her face—got out of the wrong side of the bed. I always believed being grouchy was a choice, but I felt helpless to change. Everything seemed to go wrong. Again, I asked God how this was fair. For months I had looked forward to this day, and now I was an emotional mess.

The son who was in the wedding party insisted that his new pants were too short. I tried to reason with him that they looked fine to me. He made teenage-male noises in his throat as he tugged at the offending pant legs. I looked at the clock. No time to do any altering. I tried again, but he was like a tree planted by the water—not to be moved. I dashed upstairs and flung at him the first pair of half-decent pants that matched his suit coat.

The first guests were arriving, and I still had to wash several dishes and give the counter a final wipe down. The groom's mother came into the kitchen, the picture of calmness, asking how she could help.

At that precise moment, I remembered something—the card and tags for the gifts! I flung a rag at her and told her to wipe the counters. I dashed into my closet for the wedding card. I was sure it was in my closet. A minute later I abandoned the closet to paw through drawers. I heard several more guests arrive, and I gave up the search for the card. Grabbing the gift tags and a pen, I, the writer, who wanted to tell my precious daughter and her new husband how much they meant to us, drew a blank. "Thinking of You" or "Get Well Soon" seemed fitting, but it was a wedding. "Congratulations" and "Best Wishes" were the only wedding-appropriate phrases I could think of. How lame.

The groom's mother was done wiping crumbs and looking for another way to help. "You may go out to the shop where the guests are," I replied. "But on your way out, could you go through the basement and attach these tags to the gifts, please?" I gave hurried instructions as to which tag went where. As she descended to the basement, I trotted through the house, making sure no stray tissues peeped out from under beds, and fuming that I couldn't hang the tags on the gifts myself. I loved crafting and especially gift wrapping. But what other choice did

I have? I couldn't be late for my own daughter's wedding. It was exactly like those dreams I'd had when they first were engaged, of trying to get ready for the wedding while guests were arriving and everything was chaotic. But this wasn't a dream. This was real.

I pasted a smile on my face as I started greeting guests gathering in the shop.

I had barely slept during the past several nights, and to my horror, I felt myself losing composure. I had always admired mothers of the bride as they maturely shed a few tears. Just enough tears to show attachment, but not so many that it looked unhealthy. I had certainly never seen one cry before the ceremony was well underway. The first to marry on a Friday, I thought, and the first to shed enough tears to water a garden.

My mother, who was standing nearby, noticed. "What is wrong?" she asked kindly.

"We're going to run out of food," I hiccuped. And indeed, the scaled-back guest list appeared to have an interesting science of its own. There were people arriving whom I hadn't expected, and people not arriving who were supposed to be there. Apparently in everyone's zeal to help, there had been some miscommunication.

"I'll pray that the food will multiply like loaves and fishes," my mom whispered.

"Seriously, Mom," I felt like saying. That was the kind of miracle that happened in Bible times. I believed in miracles. Just not today.

We were seated, and I didn't feel okay. The day seemed to be ruined. As the ministers filed into the council room, one of the youth boys started a song. It was unusual for a single boy to start a song during the service. I gaped and went limp.

What he was doing showed support and compassion.

Something happened deep within me. All the prayers of my friends washed over me. I had never experienced such an other-worldly feeling. If God could give this young man the courage and confidence to do the unexpected, He could do a work in me as well.

The presiding minister and deacon returned from the council room sparkling. Literally. The bishop had navy and gold glitter on his nose, and as he joined the bride and groom in marriage, the glitter sparkled. The deacon's suit coat also became alive and happy with specks of navy and gold. Our daughter had done her wedding décor with navy and gold glitter in the craft room next to the shop. To my surprise, family members had arranged benches for the ministers in that very room.

The wedding service was interwoven with sacredness. God had answered my daughter's prayer for a backyard-barbecue atmosphere. The smaller crowd had a warmth of its own.

As I sat down for the noon meal, I blinked in surprise. There, across the table in all their glory, was a row of green Melmac plates. The wedding colors were now navy, gold, and Melmac green. The doughnuts sported globs of dark-brown icing, like something you would find in a cow pasture. I tried not to laugh out loud. It didn't matter. In my zeal to prove how capable I was of planning a wedding, I had forgotten the most important thing. It was the marriage that mattered. The trimmings were nonessential.

The chicken filling, according to past weddings, had no business reaching around, but there was a whole roaster left over. I will never again doubt the prayers of my mother.

I again believe in miracles. Tradition can bring stability and order, but only God can weave two lives into one and bless the union despite circumstances. That is a miracle in itself.

At the end of the day, I had no desire to laugh at my sisters. I had a desire to hug them for always being there for me.

And no matter how much I enjoyed the day, I believe three daughters is just the right number.

A Stumbling Block to Service

Stephanie A. Leinbach

BEFORE MY SISTER told me about hospitals needing masks, I had never bothered buying or making any. Where we live in northern Indiana, wearing a mask was recommended but not required. My sister forwarded an email with a pattern and instructions. More notices flooded my inbox in the following days: "Calling all seamstresses to sew masks."

With a closet full of material and three daughters eager to sew, I was set to serve in this way.

Or was I? Questions filled my mind. "Does it matter if my material is from Goodwill?" I asked my sister. "I can't promise it came from a sanitary source."

"Oh, I wouldn't worry about that," she said. "I'm sure they will sanitize the masks before they use them."

"Well, then why is the demand so great? If they can sanitize them once, surely they could sanitize them for reuse."

"I don't know all the answers. I'm just doing what they asked. You're not obligated to sew masks; I just knew you said your girls loved to sew, and I thought they might enjoy sewing these."

Even though she didn't say it, I sensed she was tired of my questions. Maybe she sensed I was looking for excuses to appease my conscience instead of simply saying no.

I found some fabric from my stash that was not special to me and cut out a mask. I sewed it up in a matter of minutes and tried it on. It was too large. *Would it be too large for nurses?* I wondered. Next I questioned whether the material fit the tutorial's standard for tightly woven fabric. I tossed the mask and my questions aside, pursuing that avenue of service no more.

Then my husband got sick. After three days with an uncharacteristic headache, Naaman agreed I should call the doctor, but COVID-19 had shortened the doctor's hours. The earliest available appointment was for the next morning, so my husband agreed to go to urgent care instead.

He waited in the van while I walked past all the signs that screamed, "Stop! Do you have a fever? Do you have a sore throat? Do you have a cough?" At least we had no symptoms of COVID-19. But they sent me back to my vehicle, refusing to see him. These days, any out-of-the-ordinary symptoms sounded suspicious. We agreed to get a test and went through the procedure of drive-through service. After his nose was swabbed, we parked and waited for our doctor visit to be conducted by phone.

Did the doctor think she could assess the situation by hearing his voice? She did not take his blood pressure nor check his pulse. How could she say with confidence, "I don't think this is an emergency; go home and make sure you drink more liquids"?

We went home to wait for the test result. I swayed between being scared of a positive test and hoping for it. At least I would know what was wrong. They had told us the wait could be up to five days, but within twenty-four hours we received a negative result.

I then made an appointment with our family doctor. This was day five, and we needed answers. The doctor took vitals, did blood work, and sent us home with two prescriptions—ibuprofen and Tylenol with codeine. He gave us instructions to alternate the medications around the clock. He also recommended retesting for COVID-19 and urged Naaman to wear a mask. "COVID-19 is a new thing," the doctor said, "and the testing is not perfected. You easily could have been given a faulty test."

"See if Walmart has any masks," Naaman told me when we stopped to fill the prescriptions.

"You could wear the mask I made," I said.

"I will not wear a homemade mask."

I grinned because I understood his vehemence.

Of course Walmart had no masks. "We've been sold out of them for weeks," an employee said.

"I figured," I told her, "but I thought it was worth a try."

That evening my husband reacted to the pain medication, and I thought he was dying. After another night of his dreadful twisting and turning and moaning from pain, I wanted some fast answers. "If we don't get answers soon, I am going to have to be admitted to the hospital with you," I said. "Why don't we go to the emergency room? The least they could do is prove there is nothing wrong and send us home." Visions of a slow aneurysm filled my mind. His cousin had had one; maybe it was something hereditary.

The entryway door to the emergency room slid open as we approached, but the second door barred our entrance. Through the glass, we saw a secretary sitting at a little table. She pushed a button, and we conversed by intercom. I told her Naaman's symptoms, and we answered her questions: no, we had no fevers, no coughs, and no sore throats. When we told her he had a negative test result for COVID-19, she opened the door for us to enter. She reached into a box, pulled out a mask, and handed it to Naaman. She found a smaller one and handed it to me.

I wanted to grin as he slipped the homemade mask into place. It looked manly enough with camouflaged leaves on the outside; at least no one could see the teddy bear that graced the lining.

My flannel-lined mask was a snug fit. I appreciated the clean smell, but the mask almost suffocated me. We pulled our masks down over our chins and gasped fresh air anytime the doctors and nurses left the room. By the time we exited the building hours later, that clean smell was long gone. They did not ask us to return our masks.

An MRI had proven there were no tumors or aneurysms. We left with four prescriptions—three for pain and the fourth an antiviral for shingles—and I also left with a new understanding of why hospitals needed masks.

Because of someone's service, the hospital could hand me a mask. I don't know if the mask was for my protection or theirs, but someone served both of us with their duty of love. Someone did not question the validity of the need; they believed and followed instructions. Someone did not doubt that duty, but acted.

Our masks were not single-use. After we arrived home, the girls took turns trying on our masks. They continued to be a source of entertainment until Naaman's cousin mentioned her need for a mask so that she could do some shopping. I handed her his mask. "Sanitize it, and it should work," I said. "Naaman won't wear a homemade mask, and I only shop at Aldi and Walmart; they don't require them."

I wasn't the only one to have a change of mind. Naaman made a trip to Menards for some supplies. Since Menards was one of the places that had made masks mandatory for shoppers, he used one of the few work masks we had on hand for sanding. But a few days later he asked, "What happened to that mask they gave me at the hospital?"

"Oh," I said, "I gave it away. Bethann needed one, and I thought you said you would never wear a homemade mask, so I gave it to her. What about the one I made?" I found it, and he tried it on.

"This one is perfect," he said. "I might as well look as goofy as everyone else."

Does God Care?

Lavina Coblentz

"GRANDPA'S ARE COMING! Grandpa's are coming!" the children sang, dancing around the room.

"We don't know yet if they can come," my husband, Joseph, cautioned. "Don't get your hopes up too high."

Six months before, we had moved to Paraguay, South America, with our three children, Isaac, Melanie, and Cheryl. Now—at nine months and counting—our baby was due any day. Joseph's parents, John and Erma Coblentz from Iowa, intentionally planned a visit around the due date of our baby. His mother, a midwife, had delivered our other three and was hoping to do this one also.

They had purchased their tickets. But we heard borders were closing with COVID-19 restrictions in place.

My in-laws checked with the airlines and learned that all flights were still on schedule. Deciding to dare it, they boarded a plane in Kansas City on March 17, Panama bound. At Panama, the flight to Asuncion, Paraguay, still showed on the screen; a check with the ticket counter confirmed it. They waited with trepidation....

And so did we.

Please, God, make a way for them to come. Surely if You care so much about me, You'll make it possible, I prayed desperately. I did not want to have my baby at a foreign hospital, attended by nurses whose language I didn't understand.

"*Stress* makes you think Dad's have to come," my sister-in-law requoted wisely, "but *faith* reassures you they will come if it is God's will."

Half an hour before Joseph planned to leave for the airport to pick up his parents, the phone rang.

"It's Dad," he said flatly, looking at the number.

"No, it can't be!" I cried. "That means they're not coming!"

Sure enough. "Five minutes before boarding our last flight, we learned that the Asuncion airport is closing to foreigners at midnight," Joseph's dad informed him. "We need to return home."

My heart sank. Down, down, down. I resented God's plan. Did He really care about me if He allowed this?

But I forced myself to focus on His purpose. *God, what are You trying to tell me? What do You want me to learn?*

A week and a half later, Lisa Dianne—my biggest baby at a whopping nine pounds, four ounces—was born at a Russian Mennonite hospital after a short, fast labor. The nurses whisked her blue, blue form away to give her oxygen.

When my baby was returned to me, I snuggled the pink bundle close. "God," I whispered, "You *do* care! What if it had been a home birth? Would my baby girl have survived?"

But now that our baby had arrived, how would I clothe her? My in-laws had the baby clothes packed in their suitcases. God provided in ways I never dreamed of. Church sisters donated blankets, diapers, socks, and so much more. "Your baby is clothed from the missionary barrel," Joseph's sister laughingly told me.

I'm humbled to see how God cared for every detail. He used this situation to strengthen my faith in Him. Our lives are in His hands. His ways are higher than ours and past finding out.

BLESSED!

Laura Hawbaker

ON THURSDAY, MARCH 12, 2020, I went stalking the aisles of a dollar store.

The beginning of that week had been busy. My husband and I traveled, worked, attended church, went out to lunch, and kept appointments. Each day had its slated goals; Friday was the day scheduled for grocery shopping. And since we were down to just a few rolls, *toilet paper* was on the do-not-forget list.

During the week I heard rumblings about a virus called corona, but it was something that was happening in places other than Iowa. My sister was quarantined in Jerusalem, my daughter's school in Pennsylvania was closing for a few weeks, and sporting events were canceled. I remained unconcerned. My husband, Nelson, mentioned hearing about panic buying and stores having a hard time keeping shelves stocked with certain items—toilet paper in particular.

Toilet paper? No worry here. Toilet paper was on my Friday list. The main event for Thursday was to be a medical procedure on Nelson's shoulder. I went along as his driver and asked if I could accompany him during the procedure. The doctor said I could, if I wasn't afraid of needles or blood. The needles and blood weren't bad, but the chatter among the doctor and nurses was a bit disconcerting. They talked about the coronavirus, canceled sports, and empty toilet-paper shelves.

On the way home, Nelson told me to stop and buy some toilet paper. I reminded him that I planned to get groceries and household supplies the next day. He insisted. "You really should get some today; I don't think you will find any tomorrow."

My stubborn gene kicked in. I was *not* going to the store just for toilet paper. I was *not* a panic buyer. I would buy toilet paper tomorrow as planned; after all, we still had two or three rolls at home. Nelson likes to be prepared for anything, while I am more prone to see how far I can make something stretch.

We stopped at the drugstore to pick up Nelson's pain medication, and he said, "Just check out the toilet-paper selection. See if they have any, and buy some if they do."

Oh dear. The toilet-paper shelves were bare, save one lone roll. Was Nelson right? Would the grocery store be out of toilet paper tomorrow?

I took Nelson home to recuperate. Then, at his suggestion, I went to the local dollar store to look for toilet paper. As I pulled into the parking lot, I saw someone leaving the store with an armful of toilet paper.

Trying not to look like a panic shopper, I bypassed the carts and meandered toward the back of the store where the paper products were located. Yes! The shelves were moderately stocked; I even found brands that boasted more than one ply. I modestly selected two packages.

Now I had a problem. I was too embarrassed to buy only toilet paper. I didn't want to explain to the checkout clerk that we really needed this toilet paper, and that I was not hoarding. I didn't have a cart so I couldn't buy many other items, and besides, I was getting supplies tomorrow. I strolled to the home-décor aisle, looking for something to fill the blank space above the mantel.

On the bottom shelf I noticed a stack of large rectangular mottos. Flipping through them, I saw single words printed in black letters on a gray background, words like *FAMILY* and *GATHER*. Then I found the word *BLESSED*. Yes! This was what I had been looking for. Gathering up my two packages of toilet paper and my motto, I paid for my purchases.

Nelson was happy I had found toilet paper, and of course, he had been correct. When I shopped for supplies on Friday, there was no toilet paper to be found. And my motto? It was a perfect fit. I had no idea that the word *BLESSED* would become so much more than home décor.

During the next few days, weeks, and months, COVID-19 moved into my life. This microscopic virus dictated many changes to my plans and routines, and I found this unsettling. We were told by the government and health officials to stay home and stay safe. Do not gather and do not travel. Canceling church services because we might make someone sick went against everything I had been taught about church attendance. When I could not travel to be with my daughter after the arrival of her first baby, I cried and she cried. I struggled with uncertainty and despair while helping another daughter plan a wedding.

But in a way I had not previously experienced, this uncertainty drove me toward God. When apprehension began to rule my spirit, I sat on the couch with my Bible and searched God's Word, trying to make sense of all this confusion. Verses about God's faithfulness spoke to my troubled heart. This might be a novel virus to the scientists, but not to an all-knowing God. He was in control, and I could rest in Him. When I looked up from my Bible, I would see the word on the mantel. I would remind myself, "Laura, count your blessings, not your troubles."

And indeed, I was blessed. No government mandate could keep us from worshipping. Our ministers continued to preach, and technology brought their hope-filled messages right into our living room. When our congregation could not gather for spring Communion, Nelson planned a Communion service around our dining-room table with our sons, daughters-in-law, and grand-children—a Resurrection Day service we will long remember.

My daughter delivered a healthy baby girl in April. Her husband, working from home, proved to be a first-rate baby nurse. They managed quite well without an immediate visit from Grandma, and I tried to wait patiently to meet the new baby.

And what about planning a late-June wedding? This caused the most tension, and at the same time, brought great blessing. By the end of May, our governor allowed religious gatherings, which included weddings and receptions. We were thankful we were legal, yet we still agonized over decisions. My daughter and I enjoyed days of happy planning and preparing, but these days were often followed by times of anxiety and fear. This was a long-anticipated wedding and was supposed to be a fun time, not one when we discussed hand sanitizer and social distancing. How odd that this virus, while not making me physically sick, was jerking me around emotionally.

The theme for the wedding—celebrating God's faithfulness throughout life—was chosen by my daughter and her fiancé long before COVID-19 struck. How often I have glibly talked about God's faithfulness. Now it was time to celebrate and rejoice in that faithfulness, not only when life was predictable, but especially in changeable, uncertain times. I can rest in the rock-solid truth of a faithful, unchangeable God.

The wedding was just that—a celebration of God's faithfulness.

I am blessed.

Aunt Jo's Mask Factory

Sheila J. Petre

NOW IT CAME to pass that in early 2020 a new and strange pandemic called COVID-19 swept into America and changed the lives of the Petre family in Mercersburg, PA. It changed the life of their Aunt Jo, who lives just down the walk from their house in a nice little room where children like to take their chairs to sit down and visit.

Here is how life changed for Aunt Jo and the Petre family: They stopped attending church. They stopped going to school. They stopped shopping at Goodwill stores. They stopped seeing their friend Mariann.

Their friend Mariann still talked to Mama on the phone, however, and she told stories about her job—teaching English online to children in China. China was the first country in the world to spread the news about the pandemic, the novel coronavirus, which had pointed his little nose toward America as soon as he could. In China, the little children and their parents were well acquainted with the strange customs of the coronavirus and with all the Best Ways of handling him. In late March, one of the moms in China talked to Mariann about COVID-19, and she asked an interesting question. "Why aren't the people in America wearing face masks?"

Aunt Jo works at Glenwood Foods. That's one thing about her. She also likes to sew. That's another thing. And the third thing is that Aunt Jo is the best kind of aunt ever, because she is Very Skillful with working with children. You need to know these things about Aunt Jo before you can understand this story about Aunt Jo's Mask Factory.

So, we'll start with the first thing. Aunt Jo works at Glenwood Foods. The people at Glenwood Foods were very busy in those last days of March and first days of April. Many customers bought chicken and flour and toilet paper, and they talked about the coronavirus. Some of the customers wore face masks. After a while, the workers at Glenwood Foods started to talk about masks, too. "We want to do what we can to help slow the spread of the virus," they said. "Maybe we should all wear masks. But who will make them for us?"

Aunt Jo said she would do it. She brought home a disposable face mask and took it apart and thought about how it was made. She found her cutting mat and her rotary cutter, and she cut out rectangles and sewed elastic to the sides of them and pleated them and topstitched them, and soon enough, Aunt Jo had a very pretty cloth face mask. She cut some more, and she sewed some more.

She took the first mask to Glenwood Foods on the sixth of April. Glenwood's manager ordered a hundred masks. Each mask took between ten and fifteen minutes to make from start to finish. To fill her hundred-mask order, Aunt Jo was looking at sixteen to twenty hours of pinning, pressing, and sewing, all of which had to happen after she finished her work at Glenwood. And would one hundred masks be enough? Customers saw employees wearing the masks and wondered where they could get them.

Now, Aunt Jo is clever. It didn't take her long to notice that a distinct advantage of living in a house on Small Creature Corner is that she is surrounded by Small Creatures who can help her with such an easy-peasy job as cloth-face-mask sewing. The Petre children were happy to hang out in Aunt Jo's room and to help her make masks, abetted, of course, by the generous doling out of cheese-and-cracker or candy treats. With the whole family at it, Mama felt left out, so on the eighth of April, she started to help.

This was the process: Aunt Jo started with 100 percent cotton fabric, washed with salt to keep it from fading, and dried at high heat to pre-shrink it. Then someone, usually Rachael or Laurel, ironed it. For the first several hundred masks, Aunt Jo picked out the fabrics. Aunt Ralenda and Mama donated pieces from their cupboards. Glenwood employees contributed. And then, as Aunt Jo got busier, some of her friends took turns buying fabric. Grandma Lehman mailed a boxful, too. After the fabric was pressed, someone cut it into rectangles—seven inches by eight inches. Aunt Jo's friend Glenda spent hours at her house cutting fabric into rectangles.

Most of us agreed that matching was one of the most fun parts. "Does that green pasture full of white sheep match this little green print or that black plaid better? Doesn't this purple allium flower pair well with this gray paisley?"

Someone had to cut elastic to length. Sometimes, when the table was full of mask supplies, the family cut elastic on a mat on the floor. Aunt Jo said it was better to have too-long than too-short elastic, since it was easier for someone to shorten it than to lengthen it to fit. By mid-April, Aunt Jo was wearing a mask full-time at Glenwood Foods and knew the assault elastic bands could make on ears.

As the weeks passed, Aunt Jo had a harder time finding elastic. She bought it by the yard or by the spool, by the bundle and by the tangle, from local shops and seamstresses and from eBay, via one of the managers at Glenwood Foods. She paid from thirty to eighty-five cents a yard for it. Depending on the style of elastic, she asked the children to cut it anywhere from 8 ½ to 9 ¼ inches.

Mama mostly worked in the house, pinning elastic to matched patches or preparing masks for their first stitching. Then she stitched each mask on three sides, butting one mask up against another to make what the children called a "string" of masks. The longest string she sewed was seventy-five masks long and reached from her sewing machine in the front room nearly to the door of the family room. One bobbin had enough thread to sew forty-five masks.

Benjamin would run to the house and retrieve a string of masks. He snipped them apart and turned them inside out. He or his siblings pushed out the corners with scissors or a bodkin until they looked neat and even. Then Laurel ironed them flat.

Aunt Jo brought home a spool of plastic-covered twist-tie wire from Glenwood. For the first few days, the children cut two pieces of wire per mask, but before long, they realized they could make fewer cuts if they cut one long length of wire (14 ½ inches long) and folded it nearly in half, and then folded over the end of the longer side to soften the end. Eventually they discovered that if they slipped the leg of a folding chair into the center of the spool of wire, they could hold it in place and keep unspooling.

They placed their double-wire into the open side of the mask and pushed it to the top of the mask as far as they could. They pinned the wire in place.

Rachael was the primary pleater. She took the pressed, wired mask and pressed three pleats into it. She stacked the pleated masks in little piles of ten each and lined them up by the sewing machine for Aunt Jo. Sometimes she took a break to treat her siblings to a chapter or so of Story from a book kept nearby. As the weeks passed, the children liked to call and listen over the phone to Johnny Miller's story time from Christian Aid Ministries while working on masks.

After the masks were pleated, Aunt Jo made a final topstitching around the top of the mask, triple-stitching over the pleats.

By the last full week in April, the children were spending more time in Aunt Jo's room every day, and they raced to have as many masks as they could all ready for the final topstitching.

This was necessary, for as the days wore on, Aunt Jo could not keep Glenwood stocked with masks. She took off a day, then another half day. Sometimes she came home from work early. And still she could not keep up. She would take a hundred masks to Glenwood in the morning, and they were sold by lunchtime.

Other seamstresses brought in masks, too. Krislyn, the manager's married daughter, brought in nine masks one day. Aunt Jo caught Krislyn looking at her, puzzled. "What?"

Krislyn said it took her longer than she expected to sew these nine masks. How was Jolynn bringing in a hundred from a single evening? Aunt Jo showed her pictures of the little factory in action.

Nor were the children finished helping after the final topstitching was completed. They snipped the little threads and gave each mask a final pressing, and then they slipped each into a slider-bag and applied a label.

Everyone got faster and faster. But they were still not fast enough to keep up with demand. So, Aunt Jo brought in friends to help her. The children enjoyed the visitors; they provided some social interaction during those stay-at-home days. Everyone worked together to make blue masks and green ones, adult masks and children's masks, masks that were pretty and masks that were homely.

More seamstresses brought in more masks to Glenwood, attempting to keep up with the demand. The governor of Pennsylvania passed a law that after eight o'clock on Sunday evening, April 19, everyone must wear a face mask in public. The weekend leading up to that Sunday, the sales of face masks escalated; Glenwood sold over five hundred masks in a single day. Sometimes when a seamstress took a box of masks to the store, customers would mob her, sorting through her box and selecting their masks.

By now, Aunt Jo had timed herself. If the children had the masks all ready for her to sew, she and they could process forty-four masks in an hour. But they had only so many hours. Everyone was glad for the other seamstresses.

Aunt Jo and the children were pleased, though, when they realized that some Glenwood customers would sort through the Handmade Face Masks boxes, picking out masks produced by Aunt Jo's Mask Factory. Not all the other masks contained the wires, which make a mask easier to fit over a wearer's nose. And the Petre family was sure Aunt Jo's masks were the prettiest. On April 24, Aunt Jo told the children that for every ten masks they had ready for her to sew, she would give them a little bonus.

When she got home that evening, she exclaimed over the stacks of pleated masks waiting for her. "Count them," the children begged.

She counted—the whole way to sixteen stacks! One hundred sixty masks? Then Rachael told her. Each stack had twelve masks on it. One hundred ninety-two masks! Aunt Jo gave each of the children their bonus.

And the little ones? What were they doing in the middle of this factory? Keturah figured out how to unlatch Aunt Jo's door and venture out into the spring sunshine, all by herself. Stephen put together puzzles on the floor. Sometimes Benjamin helped him.

In late April, on Aunt Jo's twenty-third birthday, Mama took all the children to Glenwood Foods to see Aunt Jo and to tell her "Happy Birthday" and to buy some ham loaf for her birthday supper. That was a fun trip. The children could see all the Glenwood employees wearing masks. (They had no idea that in another two months, such a scene would no longer seem strange.) They even saw customers wearing some of the masks they had helped to make. "Did you see that old lady wearing a mask with the seed packet print?" One of the clerks wore the mask with the purple allium flowers.

And of course, the children wore masks for their shopping trip. When the family got home, they posed for a picture while wearing their masks. They were helping to slow the spread of the pandemic. The mom from China would be happy.

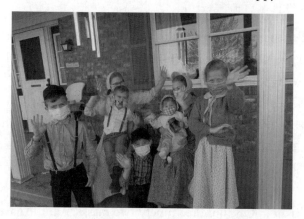

By April 26, Aunt Jo's Mask Factory had produced over 1,600 masks. How many more would it churn out? The children didn't know, but they were not tired of it yet. Besides the fun of seeing how happy people were with the masks they made, they had money they could put in their wallets. And Mama was saving some of the mask-money to buy books.

Update: The total mask count as of mid-August was 3,750. Masks were still selling, though less aggressively—between eighty and one hundred a week, depending on the selection. Despite the availability of blue surgical masks and inexpensive foreign-made masks by June and July, if Aunt Jo's mask box at Glenwood was empty, customers asked for more. Many people looked for colors that accessorized their favorite outfits. Who would have guessed that masks could become a fashion statement? In July, Aunt Jo started to make "show-your-smile" masks with clear plastic windows. These were more complicated, and the children didn't have as much opportunity to help, though they still helped to make the regular masks—when they weren't distracted by reading the new books they had earned sewing masks in the spring.

COVID-19 ... and Cancer

Linda Zimmerman

MARCH 2020 FOUND me struggling again and again with a knotted stomach. Fears of the new coronavirus, enhanced by the news media, were dogging my days. Reports of people dying with no family by their hospital beds didn't help untie the stomach knots. Would COVID-19 hit our family? Our church family? Our extended family? Our friends? There were so many unknowns concerning what this new virus could or would mean to me and to my acquaintances.

Then one night I had a dream. In the dream, a flood was raging beside me, with waves tossing high in the air. It was a terrifying dream. I cried out to my daughter, who was with me, "Hurry, we need to get to higher ground!"

On Saturday evening, March 21, our ears caught the report that the first person in our community had tested positive for

COVID. Unfortunately, it was a cancer doctor, and he had seen a number of cancer patients prior to his diagnosis. My heart went out to his patients and their families. Cancer patients on chemo, with compromised immune systems, should not be exposed to the new coronavirus. Would they be able to fight it off? This also meant the virus was now local. My struggle to ward off fears of the uncertain future continued.

As another Sunday came to an end on March 29, I wondered how long this quarantine would last. How many more Sundays would we spend at home, away from the fellowship of our church family? As I crawled into bed that night, I discovered something even more daunting—a breast lump!

I was alarmed; a lump at such a spot could very likely spell cancer for me just as it had for my mother. All sleep fled as my mind swirled with questions, fears, and possible scenarios. This meant I would need to go to town to see a doctor. COVID added a new dimension to such a doctor visit. I couldn't help but remember the cancer doctor's positive test for COVID.

If my lump was malignant, I would possibly need to go for chemo treatments. I felt trapped; COVID was closing in on me, and I was going to have to face it head-on. But I reminded myself I did not have to face COVID—or the possibility of cancer—alone.

I climbed out of bed and turned to the Psalms for comfort. My eyes fell on Psalm 16, and I jotted several verses into my journal. Verse 1, "Preserve me, O God: for in thee do I put my trust." Verse 7, "I will bless the Lord, who hath given me counsel: my reins also instruct me in the night seasons." Verse 8, "I have set the Lord always before me: because he is at my right hand, I shall not be moved."

Thus, I instructed my heart that night to trust God with my fears—fears of COVID, fears of a cancer journey, fears of the unknown in our rapidly changing world. I also reminded myself that God knew that this lump and COVID would come at the same time. If God had allowed it to be so, then I could trust Him, no matter what happened.

Psalm 61 spoke to me on Monday morning: "From the end of the earth will I cry unto thee, when my heart is overwhelmed: lead me to the rock that is higher than I." I remembered my earlier dream. Yes, where could I take my fears except to the Rock that is higher than I?

When I called the doctor, I learned that due to COVID, the clinic was only taking emergencies. They viewed my situation as an emergency and set up an appointment for the next day.

My husband, Bryan, took off work on Tuesday to take me to the appointment. Due to COVID restrictions, he ended up waiting in the parking lot. A nurse at a table inside the door asked a number of COVID symptom questions.

Some days earlier I had watched a video of a New York doctor sharing his thoughts on COVID. He had highly recommended wearing masks, thinking about the surfaces we touch, and using hand sanitizer. I was not interested in having COVID mix with this lump issue, so I had gone armed with hand sanitizer, but I had forgotten to grab one of my husband's N95 masks. The nurse had a box of masks on her table, but when I asked her for one, she refused since I did not have any COVID symptoms. When I told her I would really like to wear one, she kindly handed one to me and showed me how to wear it.

As I walked down the halls and rode the elevator, I was amazed at the stillness of the clinic, which is normally bustling with activity. I saw only one person in the hallway, a cleaning lady busy with disinfecting.

The doctor didn't seem worried about the lump but scheduled a mammogram and sonogram for the next day at the hospital.

I told my husband I would go to the appointments myself. There was no reason for him to miss work to sit in the parking lot. As I approached the hospital doors, I was confused. They were closed off with caution tape. I walked to another set of doors; they were also inaccessible. What was I to do?

I walked to the clinic next door and was told I needed to go to the emergency room doors—the only doors that were open due to COVID. As I walked around the back of the hospital, I noticed a blue "testing" tent in the parking lot, the posted "social-distancing" instructions, and red tape marking the sidewalk every six feet. I was struck by the poised and eerie feeling of everything...seemingly waiting a COVID crisis.

At the ER door, I was instructed to wait outside while using my foot to hold the automatic door open. Again, I was asked a number of COVID symptom questions. Then the nurse took my temperature before allowing me to enter. From that point on, having my temperature taken at the door became a standard procedure for all my medical appointments, no matter where they were. Masks also became a requirement to enter these medical facilities.

In the waiting room, most of the chairs were stacked off to the side to allow for social distancing. I noticed very little activity in the hospital. I thought of all the people with medical situations who should be getting attention but were being held off due to COVID restrictions.

The results from the tests that day were not what I wished to hear. The radiologist reported the lump to be a category 4B, which meant it was moderately suspicious for primary cancer. The next step was a consultation with a surgeon, and then a biopsy of the lump.

The emergencies-only ruling at the hospital and clinic were to my advantage and allowed for things to continue to move rapidly for me. The next week, I had a consultation with a surgeon who then set up an appointment for a biopsy procedure the following week. I went alone to each of those appointments. But on Monday, April 20, Bryan took me to my appointment to hear the results of the biopsy. He said, "At least I can be as close to you as the parking lot."

At that appointment, the surgeon told me the biopsy had revealed cancer. I tend to be fearful, and I had always feared cancer. Hearing of someone else's cancer diagnosis always struck fear in my heart. It was something I couldn't imagine facing, and now here I was. It was not someone else—this time I was facing a cancer diagnosis, and in the middle of a pandemic at that. In this experience of cancer diagnosis and COVID fears, I found this quote to be true, "God's grace keeps pace with what we face." God's grace is sufficient, and it will be supplied *when needed*, not the day before.

A surgical appointment was set for that week yet to remove the lump and some nearby lymph nodes for testing. This was only possible due to the emergencies-only ruling. I thanked the Lord that they considered my situation an emergency and kept things moving.

Early Friday morning, my husband dropped me off at the ER door, which was still the only door the hospital allowed people to enter. As I entered those doors, I took these verses with me. "In God have I put my trust" (Psalm 56:4). "Whither shall I flee from thy presence?...If I make my bed in [surgery], behold, thou art there....Even there shall thy hand lead me, and thy right hand shall hold me" (Psalm 139:7, 8, 10, personalized). COVID could keep my family from going with me, but it couldn't keep God and the people's prayers from going with me.

Surgery took hours longer than expected. I had a hard time coming out of surgery and ended up spending the night in the hospital. The surgeon informed me that cancer had been found in my lymph nodes and would be classed as a stage 3 unless it was found elsewhere. Testing to check for more cancer would be in the future.

On May 12, I received the call I was waiting for and yet dreading. I now had an appointment with an oncologist. The appointment was in Columbia, a two-hour drive, at Missouri Cancer Associates. Bryan really wanted to go with me to that appointment. He had not been allowed entrance to any medical facilities yet, so I doubted he'd be allowed to enter a cancer center.

The next day, I received a phone call saying I was allowed to bring one person with me to my first oncologist appointment. I don't know who was more pleased, my husband or I. Matthew 6:8 came to my mind. "Your Father knoweth what things ye have need of, before ye ask him."

My first appointment with Dr. Iliff, the oncologist, was on May 15. We found white plastic hanging over all the desks, with a little clear window for viewing the person on the other side. Below the window, a narrow slit to pass papers through completed the scene.

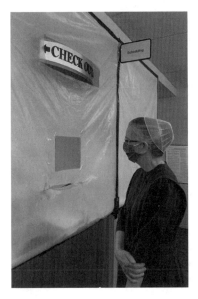

The appointment went well. I was happy to learn that my cancer had been changed from stage 3 to stage 2B. An appointment was set up for outpatient surgery to implant a port for my upcoming chemotherapy infusions.

I was back at the hospital on May 18 for a bone scan and a CAT scan to check for the presence of cancer elsewhere. As always, I needed to wear a mask and answer a number of COVID-symptom questions along with the temperature-taking ritual. There had been COVID outbreaks at a food processing plant in town, so a new question had been added. "Have you been in contact with an employee from Kraft in the last two weeks?"

The next day I had my first appointment at the George Rea Cancer Center, a division of Missouri Cancer Associates, in our local town of Kirksville. As I entered those doors for the first time, I was aware that they were doors I would be passing through many times in the next seven months. I met with Dr.

Iliff again and was grateful to hear that my scans from the day before looked clear.

The hospital now required a negative COVID test before surgery. Apprehensively, I headed to the blue tent on Thursday, May 21, and experienced my first nose swab. I had heard stories of how terrible this could be, but my experience was not unpleasant. My eyes did not even water. I was required to isolate until after surgery since they did not want me to contract COVID and bring it into the hospital. Monday the test results came back, and they were negative.

My husband again dropped me off at the hospital doors on Tuesday, May 26, this time for my port placement surgery. Things went well, and I returned home the same day.

On Tuesday, June 2, Bryan went with me to an appointment for the second time in this medical journey. Because it was my first chemotherapy infusion appointment, I was given permission to bring one person with me. How kind of the medical personnel to allow Bryan to be along for my first treatment. It was so nice to have him sitting by my side. As the chemo began dripping into my bloodstream via IV through my port, he took my hand and said, "Let's pray."

Our daughter, Treva, spent the next several days at home with me while I battled the side effects of treatment. On Saturday, she went to work, only to call home later to say she felt terrible. She had a bad headache and was hurting all over. An alarm went off in my mind. *What if she has COVID?* Since I had just had a chemo infusion, my immune system was lowered. COVID seemed determined to track me down. Did she have it or not? I did not desire to contract whatever she had—especially not COVID.

I was scheduled for lab work at the cancer center on Tuesday, and I knew I would need to say I had been around someone with COVID symptoms. I decided not to wait till that moment to find out what they would do but called in on Monday. My doctor immediately canceled my lab-work appointment and postponed my next chemo infusion for a week.

They asked that Treva get tested for COVID, so we went to a drive-through testing site. Her nose swab experience was the opposite of mine. Her eyes watered so much that she had to pull over and let me drive home. Then began the suspense—just what would we hear? A number of our church people had also come down with similar symptoms. Was it a normal flu making its rounds, or was it COVID?

Treva's results came back on Wednesday, and she was positive. I didn't know whether to laugh or cry. Some tears did squeeze out, relieving the stress that had built while we waited. The cancer center now wanted me to get tested twice. Both tests had to be negative for my chemo infusion appointments to continue.

I decided to go to the blue tent at the hospital, since I did not want to have a bad experience as Treva did at the drive-through site, but when I went the next day, I found that the blue tent was no longer in operation. I reported at the hospital door and then waited in the car until they called my cell phone. I met a nurse in a small trailer beside the hospital. The test was performed, and once again it was not unpleasant. This time a fluorescent green band was placed around my arm. I was told not to remove it until I had a negative COVID test result.

Later that day I had a disheartening phone call from a nurse at the cancer center. It seemed her main goal in calling was to fill me with fear of getting COVID. I got off the phone and dissolved into tears as I struggled to regain my footing in God once again. I reminded myself that God had not been sleeping. He knew all about it and had allowed my chemo treatment and Treva's COVID to happen at the same time; thus, I could trust Him with it all.

By evening I had enough of that bright green band around my arm. It was a depressing bit of green, a constant reminder that I might be coming down with COVID. After talking it over with my husband, I cut it off. If I needed to leave the house in the next few days, which was highly unlikely, I would patch it back together with some tape.

The phone call came on Tuesday, June 16—I tested negative for COVID. That was a miracle, considering I had been around my daughter when she was highly contagious. We later learned that one or more people had been starting with COVID at church on Communion Sunday a week and a half before. A lot of singing took place during that service, while ceiling fans moved the air around the auditorium, infecting a number of people. To social distance, I had seated myself in the entryway, but I had not worn my mask. God had protected me from getting COVID, but it was a lesson for me to be more faithful in wearing a mask in public.

Friday, June 19, I was back at the hospital for another nose swab. This time I experienced some discomfort. Thankfully, no mention was made of an armband. That procedure must have been short-lived. On Monday I heard the results. I was negative and could proceed with chemo the next day.

I dreaded this chemo infusion. I told my husband they had spoiled me by allowing him to go with me to my first appointment. Now I have to go alone to the next fifteen infusions.

Psalm 4:4 says, "Stand in awe, and sin not: commune with your own heart upon your bed, and be still. Selah." I stand in awe at times as I go onward in this cancer journey amid a pandemic. In awe of what God has done for me. In awe of what He has been teaching me through the experience. In this trial, it is my prayer that I would not sin toward God with a negative response or with a lack of trust in Him. If I can have a correct response in my heart, it will be because of God. All good and perfect things come from Him.

One COVID Sunday

Dorothy Swartzentruber

VINCENT SIGHED AND flung *Home on the Blue Ridge* onto the couch beside him. "There's just nothing to do. I wish we could see somebody again."

Annthea shut *The Secret Garden*. "Me too. It's so boring just at home all the time."

"Uh-huh!" Corwin looked up from where he was playing on his farm mat with toy equipment.

Daddy grinned at them from the recliner. "I like relaxing at home on Sunday," he teased.

"Well, yeah, I guess. But we're home all the time, and it gets so boring." Vincent stood up and stretched. "Could we go somewhere when Mama and the little ones get up from their naps?"

Daddy's eyes twinkled. "Well, Mama and I talked about something."

Corwin jumped up. "Are we going to the Empty Tomb again?" he asked. On Easter Sunday the family had driven an hour over redbud-and-dogwood-lined roads to see an Empty Tomb replica at a country junction.

Daddy shook his head. "Wait and see." He went back to reading.

"Let's go out and play pitch and catch while we wait for them to get up," Vincent suggested.

Annthea and Corwin just shrugged.

Vincent scowled. His throat felt like he'd tried to swallow a ball. What would become of his ball-playing if he couldn't practice? It had been weeks since he had seen any of his friends. And yes, weeks since he had played softball. Suddenly, he was overwhelmed with a longing for normal life again. His hands itched to feel the heft of a good bat, the powerful swing, the crack as bat connected with ball, the surge of energy as he ran for first base. "If we have a school picnic, I won't even know how to play ball anymore," he complained. He picked up his book again and flipped a few pages aimlessly.

Just then the steps creaked. Annthea leaped up and asked, "Can we go now?"

Daddy chuckled as Mama entered the living room. "You don't even know where. Are you sure you want to go?"

Annthea smiled sheepishly. "Well, I think it will be fun. Are we going to have a picnic for supper?"

Mama, looking half-asleep, sat down beside Vincent. "A picnic? I didn't even think of that."

"But where *are* we going?" Corwin stood near Daddy.

Daddy laid his book down. "Would you like to see the rapids in the conservation area?"

All three children cheered.

"What can I do?" Vincent asked. "Shall we take popcorn and baby carrots?"

"And yogurt dishes," Annthea suggested. "And graham crackers."

Mama smiled. "Sounds like you can plan a picnic yourselves! Yes, let's get it ready."

"I can make popcorn!" Vincent hurried to the kitchen and pulled out the popper. Finally, something to do. No, not playing softball, but popping corn was better than nothing.

Ideas popped in his brain as the corn popped in the kettle. "Won't there be a lot of birds in the conservation area?" he asked. "Shall I take my backpack with the binoculars and bird book in it?"

"Good idea," Mama said. "Be sure to put the camera in, too."

Half an hour later, the van rattled out the rutted lane.

"Will we see the rapids?" Rochelle asked. "Do you know where they are?"

Mama turned to look at the excited children. "We're not sure where they are, but we'll look for them. If we don't find the rapids, we'll surely see something interesting. If nothing else, the dogwoods are still blooming, and we'll have a pretty drive."

Charlotte bounced in her car seat. "I want to see rabbits, too. Will we hold them?"

Vincent chuckled and told her they were going to see *rapids*, not rabbits. Trees, fences, cows, and creeks zoomed past the van windows as the family headed north over State Road T's potholes.

Finally, they headed back a narrow gravel road. "See that blue sign on the tree, Rochelle?" Vincent pointed. "That means we're in the conservation area."

"Which way do you suppose we should go?" Daddy asked, braking as they came to a small road leading to the left.

"I have no idea," Mama said. "Try one and see where it goes."

"Hey, there's a man with a horse," Corwin said. "Maybe he knows."

Daddy got out and walked over to talk to the man. "I wish we would just get there," Corwin said. "I'm bored with sitting in the van. You should have brought a book along, Mama. Then you could read to us."

"I wish you would read *The Wheel on the School* again, Mama," Vincent said. "That was such a fun book."

Mama turned and smiled at them. "It was fun to read that book. But I'm having fun looking at all the pretty trees. Aren't you? If I were reading, I couldn't see the scenery."

Daddy got back in. "We can see the river from either of these roads, but the rapids are to the left."

They turned left and the road, cut into the sides of the hills, grew steeper and narrower. Mama gasped as the van rumbled over a washboard of potholes.

Daddy grinned at her. "We'll be fine," he said, speeding up to climb the next hill.

And then they could see it, a ribbon of brown rolling water up ahead. The road disappeared into the water as if a monster had gobbled it up. Water lapped lazily at the edge of the road, looking as if the monster wanted to eat more road when it got hungry again.

"We *have* had a lot of rain," Daddy said. "No wonder the river is flooded." He parked the van where a trail ran off to the right. "Well, let's go see what's here."

As they walked toward the river, Annthea shrieked. "A snake!"

Vincent ran close to the black snake sunning himself on the road. The snake reared up, its tongue flicking in and out.

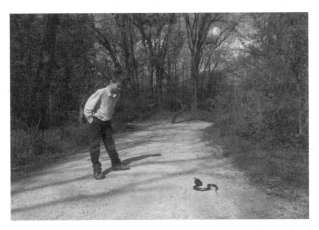

Corwin, Rochelle, and Charlotte howled with laughter as Vincent flicked his tongue in return, trying to do it as fast as the snake. Then he hopped at the snake, and it whipped into the grass. Vincent leaped after it.

"Don't!" Mama called. "There's poison ivy in there."

Vincent stopped short. Sure enough, glossy three-leafed plants stood close together as if to say, "If you dare enter our territory, we'll make you suffer for it."

They couldn't walk far on the road, nor could they see the rapids, because they were hidden under the floodwater. "Well, there isn't much to see or do here," Daddy said. "Let's go back and see what's down the other road."

When the road dropped steeply around a curve, Daddy parked the van next to a bridge across a shallow forty-foot-wide gravel-bottomed creek.

"Oh, look, children!" Mama pointed to their right. "See those cute little waterfalls!"

Vincent ran along beside the series of pools and waterfalls into the edge of the trees. He tossed a stick into the rushing stream, where it whirled and then zipped over the edge of the nearest falls. He raced the stick down to the rest of the family.

The girls tried walking across a little dam of sticks and leaves, and Corwin climbed a small strip of rocks between two falls.

"Careful, don't fall in," Mama called. "I didn't bring extra clothes for anybody."

Daddy grinned. "They would dry fast in this heat. And it's shallow; they'll be fine."

Vincent jumped down over the bank to land on an island and then leaped over the gushing water to the opposite bank. "'Look out, all ye mortals in Shora!'" he yelled as he backed up for his next run.

Everybody laughed as they recognized his quote from *The Wheel on the School*.

"Are you Janus?" Corwin asked. "But you have both your legs, and I don't see any sharks in here."

After enjoying the little stream awhile, the family walked to the bridge. They sat on the low cement ledge and watched the water flowing underneath them.

"I see Flotsam and Jetsam!" Charlotte cheered when the water swept a few sticks and leaves under the bridge. Everyone laughed again; that was another phrase from *The Wheel on the School*.

"There's more Flotsam and Jetsam." Rochelle pointed.

Daddy walked across the bridge and onto the stones near the water. He picked up a stone and skipped it over the water, past the rest of the family.

Vincent raced over to Daddy and collected his own handful of shale chips.

"They don't skip as well on running water as on still water," Daddy told him.

Vincent and Daddy competed to see whose stone would skip farther. Mama sat on a rock near Daddy and tried to capture the skips with the camera. The others hurled stones and rocks into the water, enjoying the splashes.

Finally, Daddy stood up. "Shall we see if we can get onto that gravel bar?" He pointed up the river. "I'm pretty sure there's a trail."

Whooping, the children scampered ahead. Mama followed them. Vincent scanned the weeds along the bank and spotted the trail. Grass rustled past his arms as he dashed through the growth toward the river. Leaping over a strip of mud, he landed on the gravel bar near a sycamore log. "Come on, Corwin, let's go exploring!"

"Oh, listen to that water running," Mama said as she sat on the log. "I could stay here all week and listen."

Everybody started collecting pretty rocks.

"This one must be a dinosaur tooth."

"And this one looks like a piece of petrified lung, see?"

"Oh, Mama, I found a heart!"

After admiring many rocks and swinging on a vine hanging from a large tree branch and throwing more rocks into the rippling water, the family reluctantly left the gravel bar. They sat on the grass near the little waterfalls to eat their picnic.

Mama looked up at the trees overhead. "I thought there'd be a lot of birds here. We have so many more at home this spring than usual. But I don't think I've heard a single one here in the conservation area."

Daddy cocked his head. "Huh. You're right. I wonder why they're not here."

"They're probably all at our feeder," Corwin said with a grin.

Later, as the family got back into the van, the baseball-stuck feeling grew in Vincent's throat again. *This was fun, but I still wish we could see somebody!*

As they headed home, the family watched the sunset and counted deer in fields and ditches.

"Shall we drop in at church and pick up the church mail?" Mama suggested.

Daddy agreed. Minutes later, he slowed the van to turn in at church. Vincent noticed a car near the porch.

"Hey, somebody else is here!" he exclaimed. Hope rose in his heart and the baseball shrank instantly. "But whose car is it?"

It was Scott and Rosalie, also getting their church mail. The family scrambled out of the van, eager to visit with friends from church. After saying hello, Annthea and the younger children ran to the basement for balls and brought them up to the lane to play.

Scott and Rosalie stood beside their car, and Daddy and Mama stayed beside the van, honoring the six-feet-apart restriction. Vincent stood beside Mama, listening to the adults visit. He looked across the lane to the ball field. Empty. Deserted. The baseball was back in his throat, bigger than before.

"It bothers me to see that lonely ball field," he whispered.

Mama gave him a sympathetic smile. "I believe you."

The men were discussing Scott and Rosalie's planned move to Oklahoma when an ancient Mercedes slowed on the highway and pulled in. It stopped near Scott's car, and a bushy-headed man got out of the back seat.

"Hey, good evening, guys. I'm homeless and my car ran out of gas five miles back there"—he waved to the east—"and these good people picked me up and will take me to the gas station. But I don't have any money, and they don't either. Would you help me out with some gas money?"

Scott and Daddy exchanged fleeting glances.

"So where is your car?" Scott asked.

The man waved his hand. "Oh, back there about ten miles."

Vincent wanted to snicker. *That car must be backing up pretty fast if it could drive five miles in a half minute. Out of gas, all right!*

Scott cocked his head. "So where do you live?"

The man gave a vague answer. And then, after claiming to be a Christian, he started rattling off John 14.

Scott and Daddy looked at each other again. "I don't have any cash with me," Daddy said.

Scott thought a moment. The man began quoting Bible verses again. Shrugging a little, Scott pulled out his wallet and handed the man a bill. "Be sure you use it for gas," he instructed.

"Oh, yes! Of course!" The man launched into another Scripture recital as he backed toward the open car door.

A grin played over Scott's face. "Funny thing is, we're homeless too. Our place here is sold, and we haven't finished the paperwork for our place in Oklahoma."

It was getting dark, and Daddy soon told the children to put the balls away. Scott and Rosalie left, and the family headed for home.

"That man—do you think he was truly homeless?" Vincent asked.

Daddy shrugged. "He could be. We can never tell. Jesus told us to give to those who ask of us, so it's right to give if we can. Our money is His anyway, so He will take care of the details."

At home, Daddy checked the emails.

Vincent plunked onto the couch and listened as Daddy read an email about COVID restrictions in Africa and Latin America, where people were going hungry because of police-enforced lockdowns. Many people feared they would starve. Some people were allowed to go only a few hundred feet from their houses, and others were hardly allowed that. Everyone was quiet for a minute when Daddy was done.

"Imagine being stuck in a little apartment, and not having a yard to play in or places to spend time outside," Mama said. "Imagine being homeless and having no place to go."

Vincent raised his eyebrows. "You know what?" he said slowly. "We really have it good. We have a home, we have nice places to be outside, and we even got to see somebody from church today." This time, there was no baseball in his throat.

Flour Shower

Regena Weaver

FORGIVE ME; I didn't mean to be a hoarder.

When I first encountered empty shelves at the grocery store, I was mostly amused, because they weren't in the aisles where my needs lay. As stories circulated about major hoarding and ridiculous prices for necessities, I became incredulous.

But as weeks rolled by, I got used to the signs limiting items in short supply. I didn't mind, since that was better than empty shelves. Besides, my habit of keeping essentials stocked stood me in good stead. I had found toilet paper on sale just before the pandemic, so I had sufficient on hand to last until the supply caught up with the demand. I could live with the grocery store's limit of two gallons of milk—the corner store just down the road had no limits, and I could finish filling my needs there. It wasn't a time to price shop necessities.

Then came the day I left several grocery stores without finding a single bag of all-purpose flour. I wasn't desperate yet; I had an almost-full bag of whole wheat flour in my pantry cupboard. That evening my husband and I searched online for a flour mill that would ship flour, but flour was out of stock everywhere we checked. The following week, I thanked God as I snatched up the last big bag of flour on the shelf at our small local grocery store. Never mind it cost twice what the store-brand bags did at the bigger stores in the city; it was still a reasonable price for name-brand flour.

Then our friend came to visit.

Our relationship with Mike spans a decade. Since he no longer lives locally, his grandfather status in the family has survived via phone contact and the occasional visit.

Now, in the middle of the pandemic, he came.

Early Sunday morning, he called from his motel to announce that he was stopping at the grocery store before coming to our place for breakfast. Was there anything we needed? I was torn between my Mennonite upbringing regarding Sunday observance and knowing he would be delighted to do a favor for us. At the same time, I knew he would go shopping whether or not we shared a need. After a brief deliberation, I suggested that a couple of gallons of milk would postpone my need for shopping.

It should not have surprised me that he arrived laden with multiple yellow shopping bags. My requested two gallons of milk had morphed into four, and had been joined by Rice Krispies and marshmallows (a broad hint he would appreciate some Rice Krispie bars), ice-cream popsicles, and white sugar.

"I couldn't find any white flour, but I got you some whole wheat flour." He gestured toward the three bags my son had carried in for him.

My husband and I exchanged amused glances as we surveyed our Sunday-morning groceries. He shrugged. What else could we do?

That afternoon, our restless guest headed out to spend time with his daughter. Several hours later he returned, again carrying yellow bags. With the tenacity of a bulldog, he had returned to the grocery store to see whether they had restocked the all-purpose flour. They hadn't. But that didn't keep him from buying flour. He got one of each specialty flour that was on the shelf: corn flour, self-rising flour, chickpea flour. Thanks to Google, I suppose I'll be able to figure out how to use four pounds of each of these.

The next morning before breakfast, he went shopping again. My husband tried to talk him out of it, assuring him we would be fine for a while with what he had already brought us. But it would be as easy to silence a rooster as convince Mike otherwise when he has latched onto an idea. Hoping to distract him from his quest for flour, I suggested that a few bricks of cheese would fill a need. It didn't work, though I appreciated the cheese he added to his cart.

He was positively glowing when he returned. "I found you some flour! I got the last seven bags!"

I almost choked on my coffee. What about the people who arrived at nine thirty, hoping for a chance at the new skid of flour? I wasn't sure whether to laugh or blush at the ludicrous sight of my growing pile of flour.

"How long will that last you?" my benefactor asked later that day, looking with satisfaction at the spoils. "A couple of weeks?"

I assessed the rows of five-kilogram bags of Robin Hood lining the kitchen wall. "It will depend on whether I bake my own bread. But it will definitely last for quite a while. Thanks to you, I won't be looking for flour anytime soon." I saw no need to explain that I had already offered a bag or two of flour to a few close friends. Of course, our household could put it to good use in the months ahead, but it salved my conscience to offer it, in case someone had been disappointed due to my unintentional accumulating.

There is one consolation. With social distancing in effect, I won't have someone unexpectedly showing up at my house. I would hate to explain my sudden penchant for hoarding.

Catching the Virus

Luke S. Martin

"HEY, LUKE, CAN you come here a bit? We need to talk." Titus beckoned me toward the cluster of men gathered at the back of the auditorium after the close of Wednesday prayer meeting. Faces were intent as they discussed the latest news.

"Did you hear that the president closed all the schools today?" Titus asked.

"I heard a few rumors, but nothing definite," I replied.

"Well, this is for real," Jheyson said. "They're trying to get a handle on this coronavirus outbreak. As of noon today, the president has closed all schools in Peru—public and private— by supreme decree."

"So are we actually going to close down, too?" I asked. School had started only yesterday. I was excited about spending the next nine months with my twelve students. Must we lay it all down so soon?

"Even if you and I aren't worried about catching the virus," Titus said, "it's not just about us. Think what the neighbors would say if they see our children coming to school every day. The whole nation is petrified of COVID. Plus, this is a government mandate. I think we'd better close school."

And so, we did. My plans and preparations—my identity, even—were that quickly tossed into the ditch of uncertainty and abnormality. All over a microscopic virus that modern medicine was powerless to stop.

The next several days, changes bombarded our lives. Our deacon's family, who for months had been planning a trip to the States, had their travel plans dashed only two days before the departure date. A Mennonite family, returning to Canada after visiting family in Bolivia, arrived in Lima only to discover they could not continue their journey. I drove to the airport and brought them to our community.

On Tuesday, March 17, the lockdown took effect. Only vehicles with police authorization were allowed on the road. Huaral turned into an eerie ghost town overnight. Most stores closed. The few frightened people on the street avoided each other and tried to hide their fear behind their face masks. Police patrolled the streets, forcing stores to close if they didn't follow the quarantine regulations. Shortly after six o'clock every evening, police trucks and motorcycles roared through town, making sure everyone obeyed the curfew.

Wednesday came and went with no prayer meeting. On Sunday we stayed home and listened to a recorded sermon.

I guess we can put up with this for a week or two. Or even three, if it comes to that. We'll do our part to keep from spreading this virus. And then we can hit resume and make up for lost time. Or so I thought.

For months, our church had been reaching out to the Venezuelans in our area. More than half a million had arrived in Peru over the past several years. Five thousand of those had settled in our local town. We helped the newcomers with lodging money, food, blankets, and medical assistance. Slowly they were establishing themselves. But then the COVID lockdown came and knocked their feet right out from under them.

We called an outdoor members' meeting to discuss how to respond. "The situation could get bad, fast," warned Jheyson. "The Venezuelans will be the first ones to suffer. Most of them are earning just enough each day to survive. With businesses closed and few people on the street, they won't have any way to earn a living. I think we'd better get ready to help a *lot* of people."

"So what can we do?"

"I think we need to focus on basic needs, like groceries. There is no way we'll be able to help everybody with all their needs. But if we focus on the necessities, hopefully we'll be able to ease their pain."

We didn't have to wait long to see just how many folks would be coming for help. On Thursday, March 26, I joined several other volunteers in our now-unoccupied church auditorium. The day before, Titus had brought a pickup-load of rice, lentils, potatoes, and oatmeal. We divided the goods into family-sized bags. Pop hauled the bagged goods to the distribution center a quarter mile away.

After Pop returned from one of his trips, he said, "Luke, you should go down to the distribution center and take some pictures. There are crowds of Venezuelans milling around down there." I grabbed my camera—and my recently fabricated face mask—and rode down. As I turned the corner, I was stunned. Dozens of people stood in line on the sidewalk. A row of moto-taxis lined one side of the street. Several car taxis waited on the other side. Even a bus was parked there.

Inside the distribution center, Jheyson registered each party. Ernest, with several helpers, oversaw the distribution of groceries.

"Jheyson, we've got to do something about that huge crowd of people outside," I said. "With the rest of town so quiet, we are attracting way too much attention. You know what the police do with people who break quarantine rules." We had heard the story about a neighbor boy who had been hanging out with some of his friends in the street one evening. The police found him, hauled him off to the police station, and made him do military exercises all night long.

"Don't complain to me," Jheyson said. "Go do some crowd control yourself."

Pop and I ordered the people to spread out. We asked some of the crowd to wait on the other side of the street. "At least it's a little better," I said, returning inside to help hand out the goods.

A few minutes later, I glanced out the window. "Here come the police," I exclaimed. "Jheyson, you go talk to them."

"What's going on here? Is everything okay?" the officer inquired.

Jheyson briefly explained our mission.

"So you all are okay? No one robbed you?"

"No, we're fine. We've not been robbed. We're just overwhelmed with all these people coming."

"Glad to know you're all right. We received several calls that you were being robbed. But, yes," agreed the officer, "you need a better system. Don't have so many people come at one time."

That day we handed out groceries to almost two hundred families.

The next day, even more people came. We worked hard. By evening, we had bagged nearly two tons of groceries, served 275 families, and logged ninety man-hours.

On Saturday, we called another meeting and gathered in my classroom. If we were going to survive the escalating needs, we would have to organize ourselves better. Someone needed to buy groceries almost every day. Someone needed to bag groceries almost every day. Several needed to help hand out groceries almost every day. And someone needed to register the recipients almost every day. I drew up a list on the whiteboard to help us visualize the needs and to decide which brother could best fill each need. By the time we had finished, I had written nearly everybody's name on the board.

The Venezuelans weren't the only ones benefiting from this aid project. It pulled our brotherhood together when social distancing and quarantine threatened to pull us apart. Working for the good of others gave us purpose in the midst of uncertainty.

Throughout April the distribution continued to increase. Our church house turned into a packing house; we pushed all the benches to the front and spread out up to a ton and a half of potatoes at a time to sort and bag. Often, as many as ten volunteers worked together bagging out potatoes, rice, and lentils. Rather than having all the Venezuelans come to our distribution center, we began delivering to over thirty drop-off points in town.

Through May and into June, the grocery distribution maintained a steady rhythm.

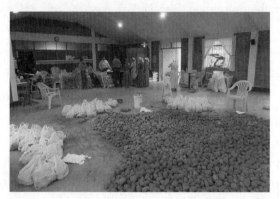

Church house turned packing house

So far none of us had gotten sick with the dreaded virus. If anything, we had suffered less sickness this winter than usual. Was it because we were wearing face masks and disinfecting regularly with alcohol? Or was it simply God's protection over us? We shuddered to think what would happen if COVID swept through our church. Likely, the aid project would have to be shut down.

If anybody in the community was being exposed to germs, it was us. We visited groups all over town. We handed groceries to poor families who emerged from dinky alleys. We handed out groceries along the street, attracting attention from far and near. At one drop-off point, such a large crowd had gathered that the police threatened to break up the group and jail the coordinator. That time, we met over one hundred needy people, who eagerly held out their backpacks and old market bags to receive goods for their family. What a perfect environment for germs to spread.

Then around the middle of June, as quarantine laws subsided and businesses opened again, we cut back on the grocery distribution and began focusing on other areas. Many Venezuelans had medical needs. The government hospitals were only seeing COVID patients and emergencies, while private clinics charged far more than any Venezuelan could afford. We also received many requests for blankets and clothing to combat the cold weather. To help us sort through all these needs, we decided to require that any Venezuelan requesting aid first needed to fill out a questionnaire.

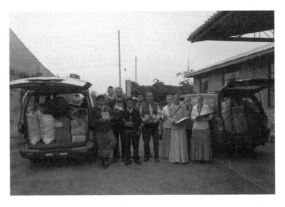

Distribution Crew

Once again, we gathered to discuss the aid project.

"Ernest," I said, "you mentioned that on the questionnaires many Venezuelans requested a visit for spiritual help. How are we going to fulfill those requests?"

"Good question. So far we have done very little."

"It seems to me we have before us a tremendous opportunity. These folks have lived through lots of tough experiences.

Now they want a visit and spiritual support, which is even more important than groceries. God has put an open door right before us!"

"Luke, I agree with you," Jheyson said. "But we are all so busy already. How can we add another activity to our program?"

"Could we arrange an afternoon or two a week when whoever has some time can go visiting? I think it would be worth cutting back on some of our other aid activities to have time to do this."

"Oh my, we need Daniel here," Pop lamented. Daniel, our minister, and his wife had gone to the States at the end of February and still hadn't been able to return.

"It's pointless to wish for more folks to come and help," Ernest said, "with the borders closed for at least several months yet. This coming week, let's see if we can arrange a few visits. I know Silvio would be glad to help. Any of the rest of you that have a free afternoon, let me know. Let's see what we can do."

Silvio was to prove an invaluable asset to the work. A Venezuelan himself, he had arrived in our area a year and a half ago. He was in instruction class and his commitment to Christ was obvious.

Over the next several weeks, we made many new friends as we visited in the homes of our Venezuelan contacts.

Carmen struggled to relate to her daughter-in-law. And who wouldn't? Carmen lived with her son and daughter-in-law and their five children in a one-room apartment. The family listened attentively to the preaching and counsel we shared with them on the rooftop of their apartment complex. While Carmen's son had some Bible knowledge, the rest had only a nominal Catholic understanding.

One young man was frightfully ignorant of eternal truth.

"Do you know who Jesus is?" Silvio asked him.

A blank expression met his question.

"Who is God?" Silvio tried again.

The young man creased his brow as if trying to remember the correct answer to a Sunday school quiz from ten years ago. "Isn't He like the one who made the earth and stuff?"

"What an opportunity!" Silvio told us later. "We have folks right on our doorstep who have never heard the Gospel. A fire is burning in my bones to get this message out. Let's get out there and preach wherever we can. Young men, we need you to help! We have the message that these folks need to hear. We've been sharing material goods with them. Now their hearts are wide open to receive spiritual goods as well. It's like God is giving us the perfect excuse to preach Christ to them."

Fernando and Jessica were a young Christian couple with a young daughter. Fernando told us he had been seriously studying the Bible and seeking the Lord during the pandemic. "So many 'Christians' do not follow Christ at all," Fernando said. "We are lonely and long for fellowship."

Another family we visited consisted of two grandma sisters and their descendants. Rarely had we found Venezuelans so zealous for the Lord. These former Baptists passionately evangelized their neighbors. They pled with us to hold a service for them and their neighbors. So, one evening a small group gathered in the alley in front of their house. We sang, and then I preached about bearing the yoke of Jesus. We were all blessed, even though very few neighbors attended. Soon we started a weekly Bible study with the family.

María, a humble mother of three children, told us she is reading all the literature we give her. She is searching for something in our belief that she does not agree with, but so far, she hasn't found anything. Her husband puts in long hours to support his family—he often gets home after midnight.

This modest María shared her testimony with us. "I'm a Christian and was baptized when I was nineteen years old. My husband is also a Christian. My husband is my head, and his head is Christ. I don't go out preaching a lot to the neighbors, because I believe my life needs to be my testimony. My life needs to be the salt that draws others to the Gospel."

We took groceries and blankets along for one poor family that had just arrived in the area. "Do you have your own Bible?" we asked the mother as we finished up the visit. She shook her head. "Well, here is one for you." With a smile, Judith handed her a shiny paperback Bible.

"For me?" the woman stammered. "Oh, how I have longed to have my own Bible! Thank you! *Thank you!* Of all the things you've given me, this Bible is the most precious." Her glowing eyes were more than reward enough.

Most Venezuelans received us graciously and thanked us for coming. Occasionally, however, we met with resistance. As several of us finished up a visit one afternoon, a Peruvian fellow came walking up. After asking what we were doing there, he turned to me. "Why are you standing here talking to me without your mask on?" he growled. To oblige him, I pulled up the mask I had pushed down to converse. He continued to fuss about our infraction. He claimed he was a lawyer and kept asking who we were and why we were here. My discomfort grew. Soon I eased over to Silvio. "Let's get out of here," I whispered.

As we told our hosts goodbye, the intruder barked out, "Hey, what did you say your name is?" I turned to see him talking on his phone. "Lucas Martin de Huando. Look him up there and see what you can find on him."

Our apologetic hostess walked back to the car with us. "That shady character is a brother to the owner of the house we're renting. He thinks he can run the show around here."

In the car, I asked Silvio, "Did you see he was talking on his phone?"

"Really? I doubt he actually was talking to anybody. He saw you were afraid of him, and he was manipulating you. Lucas"—Silvio turned to me with that wise, fatherly look in his eyes—"dealing with opposition like this is part of evangelizing. The devil is not happy. We are in a spiritual warfare."

I knew he was right. Still, I breathed a sigh of relief that evening once I was safely back in the compound, inside our little haven of rest with my precious family. And that evening, seated at the head of the table with my family around me, I prayed that God would help me not to give in to fear, but to keep on spreading the Good News.

The next day at our staff meeting, we discussed our experiences of the week. Silvio thanked all of those who had helped with the visitation. "I am so happy to see the virus spreading!"

We looked at Silvio quizzically.

Silvio chuckled. "Yes, the passion to preach Jesus to the people is contagious. And I praise the Lord that you all are catching this virus! People are hearing the Gospel. Even if only one comes to Jesus, it will be worth it all."

How COVID-19 Reset My Mindset

Lucinda J. Kinsinger

IVAN AND I HAD been married for a little over three months when COVID hit the news. The governor of Maryland issued a stay-at-home order just after we passed our four-month mark. When we married, I had moved from a close-knit family and church community in Wisconsin, so spending long hours alone on the days Ivan worked away from home made me feel bored, lonely, and trapped. I would call my mom sometimes or walk across the yard for a brief visit with Ivan's parents, who were in their eighties and liked the company. But without church, writers' events, and other social interaction to keep me occupied, my mind felt like a sausage ready to burst its casing.

A friend told me her lifestyle hadn't changed all that much since quarantine. Seeing everyone else panic over the social isolation that was normal for her validated what she had been feeling—a sort of crazy-making loneliness, a need for friends.

Yes, I agreed with her. Human creatures aren't meant to be alone.

But as my whirling mind slowed and the dust settled, I realized some of the benefits of COVID. Because I didn't have other events to fill my calendar, I went with Ivan more often on his hauling trips, and those times turned out to be excellent opportunities for honest and natural conversation. With only each other for companionship and entertainment, our bond strengthened exponentially. Several months of intense togetherness at the beginning of a marriage to build a strong foundation? I highly recommend it.

Here are some more things the crony-virus (as my husband likes to call it) taught me:

Busyness is not as necessary as I thought it was. Yes, I missed church, and I was truly disappointed when visits from my Wisconsin family had to be postponed. But I wouldn't have wanted to give up the quality time Ivan and I shared. Time with family and church is important, of course. But how much of it do we need? What about time for events and conferences and Christian ministry and socializing with friends? How much busyness is too much? Another way of asking this: How important am I? I tend to feel that if I don't take part in social and ministry events, both I and those around me will miss out on something valuable. But is that a conceited way to view my participation? Perhaps just as many helpful words will be spoken, just as many people encouraged, just as many souls won for Jesus if I stay home more often. I began to think so, after I had practiced it awhile.

God's acts are more powerful than anything humanity can achieve. I do not mean to say He manufactured the virus for our punishment, but that He controls the natural world and chooses to allow or not allow what happens in it. And it turns out that the processes of the natural world are much more powerful than the best or the worst humans can enact. Think about it. For years we've feared terrorists and wars and mass shootings and nuclear blasts. But the one thing that brought the world to its knees was a disease. Perhaps people had a role in creating it by providing conducive conditions, but the actions of the disease itself—the way it spread from person to person and skipped between countries like a calf jumping hillocks—are beyond our puny human control.

The world is smaller than it used to be. In the 1300s, the bubonic plague traveled on a fleet of "death ships" from Asia to Europe, where it killed a third of the population. Still, huge swaths of the world remained untouched. In today's easy-travel culture, almost every country was affected by the coronavirus. I have never before seen the whole world so riveted to one thing as they were to this disease. The virus is not a good thing, but it has been eye-opening and rather refreshing to see how connected we all are.

God still reigns. In any situation, under any circumstance. In that we can rest. Many people felt high levels of anxiety during COVID-19, as evidenced by the empty shelves in the grocery stores where toilet paper and bread and milk, and hand sanitizer used to be. While some preparation can be a good thing, God's children need never panic buy, whether in a physical or spiritual sense. His grace is sufficient every day. He is able to form in us deeper faith and stronger relationships from even the worst circumstances in life. *Especially* from those.

From Schoolteacher to Big Sister

Megan Byler

IT IS APRIL 16 and nearly a month since I had to leave the job I love to let my students homeschool. I had so many plans for those last few months of school—program practice, stargazing, perfecting penmanship. But I had to give them all up.

At first it was hard to accept; I wanted to go back to my little school so much. But then it struck me: *This must be God's plan for me right now, and only in the center of His will would I be truly happy.* I firmly repeat this to myself on days when it is not easy to let go of what I wish I could be doing.

Having time to do whatever we want is one of the biggest blessings of this lockdown life. With everyone around, Mom started an ambitious backyard makeover—digging paths, enlarging the flower beds, planting a boxwood border, and painting the outside of our house. Right now it wears tan and gray, the latter being the new color. As fast as Dad puts up siding on his free days, we show up behind him with the bucket of paint.

Then the doors begged for a face-lift. We ladies went on a hunt and discovered the perfect color to go with gray siding— Hint of Cherry Pink. We asked the man of the house for his opinion. He looked unsure, but being such a nice man, he agreed to a trial run. We solemnly promised to try the new color on the back door first.

I found it's a good idea to start a world-changing project like this when you have to babysit your little siblings. They all gathered around, wide-eyed and wanting to help. Presto! Perfect behavior. We viewed the door from several angles in the backyard and decided the new color was for keeps. Even the man agreed.

I stained the wood walls of Dad's new office one Monday—a good Monday project that wouldn't require too much concentration. But when I climbed the ladder to finish up, it took a happy little scoot, and I was left behind, leaping backward from a wave of stain pouring from the can. Thankfully, Dad was home and came running to help when he heard my screams. Dads are so good at things like that.

Having time has brought more blessings:

More time to take walks with my little brothers, Conner and Quinn. They splash mightily through the puddles. And I still get a childish thrill from looking into the puddles to see an endless world reflecting down, down, down.

More time to sew matching dresses with Mom—thanks to Tiffany, who found the polka-dot material for us back when we could still shop freely.

More time to cook and bake again. My family was sure that teaching made me lose housekeeping skills. They seemed surprised to find out I could still make supper. The problem is, now that I have time to do this, I feel like I'm about twelve years old again. Back then when I planned a supper, I would pick all the exciting recipes. Those recipes were a grocery list in themselves. Now, sitting at home and looking at all these cookbooks makes me want to do that again. Maybe it's good that a ban on nonessential travel keeps me from frivolous trips to the grocery store.

More time to help Tiffany and Travis with the spring clean-up. We signed up to mow the lawn at a cemetery this summer, but I thought I wouldn't be able to help until May, when school ended. We spent two days there last week, raking, raking, raking. It was nice to do some hard work again, after all of our lazy days at home. The only problem on the job is that the cemetery has gravestones large enough for a fifteen-year-old brother to hide behind. Tiffany and I screamed loud enough to satisfy him for a long time.

More time to plan more picnics. We ran out of marshmallows on the last one, long before Travis was ready. He was so desperate for marshmallows that he roasted a whole string of mini ones; there's not much left of them once they've been through the fire. Bronwyn and I decided to sleep in our wee tent by the campfire that night. I had forgotten how much fun it is to lie in a sleeping bag and listen to the fire crackle, hear the train whistle as it passes through Chatham, and see sparks dance past the tent window.

We've had so much more family time simply because there *is* time. Tonight we ran out to the park after supper to play softball and tennis. Tiffany and I discovered how much we like playing tennis and decided to do it often this summer.

I had time to have an art class with my little siblings one day. The Plan was to fill balloons with those squishy water beads and knot them shut to make stress relievers. The Problem was getting them in there. We knocked over the can of water beads in the process and had a beautiful, sparkling mess on the floor. With glee, Quinn hopped down and smashed them flat. Doing an art project with siblings isn't much different from teaching an art class at school.

Despite the moments when I miss teaching my ten little people and I wonder when the pandemic will end, I feel so blessed because I have all this time with the people I love. God's adventures are always worth saying *yes* to.

The Strangest Funeral I Never Was At

Marlene Brubacher

I KNOW ABOUT funerals; I've been to half a hundred. I was raised in a bishop's house, and I often helped with preparations backstage. In old times, as soon as we got news of a death, we began preparing to print funeral programs and memorial cards at the small printshop in our backyard. In old times, as soon as we got news of a death, we cooked lots of food. We live in a semi-isolated community in the North, where large church functions involve company from all over, so funerals usually meant every home from the congregation hosted overnight guests. In old times, there were lots of phone calls and food-committee meetings and trustee plans and bustling.

Not this time.

Cleason and Mary Martin, our elderly bishop and his wife, loved God and people—all people. Their faces lit up when they saw someone to visit with. It is no wonder they had been chosen to move north in the mid-1970s to pioneer a church in the rocks and muskeg of Mine Centre, Ontario. Nor is it surprising that after most of their family was grown, their love for Kingdom expansion led them to mission fields in Guatemala, India, and Bulgaria. In the spring of 2020, Mary learned that her cancer was back after having been in remission for more than a year. Two weeks later, she died.

In old times, Sister Mary's funeral would have been attended by six or eight hundred people. But in May 2020 we were still frozen in our locked-down community, where no one came and no one went. So though my parents sat down with the family to plan the service, and though we printed the funeral program and memory cards as usual, and though sisters from church sent meals to the family and prepared sack lunches for them to pick up on the funeral day, and though my brother Nathan mowed the church lawn during the grave digging, and though my brother Galen spent hours planning the technology necessary for a virtual funeral, I hardly realized there was going to be a funeral, until Wednesday night after work when I went to the drive-in viewing.

It was an odd, odd viewing. Ontario's limit per gathering was five people, but we were generously allowed ten for funeral proceedings. Ten people does not feel generous, however, to Mennonites, whose friends are measured by hundreds and thousands. We all stayed in our vehicles around the perimeter of the parking lot, waving at beloved church friends whom we had not glimpsed for months. Then we took turns, ten at a time, with requisite two-meter (six-and-a-half-feet) spaces between families, to enter our church lobby where the casket sat.

None of Mary's family stood by the casket, and the forsaken foyer echoed strangely. I remembered how Mary had been the first person to greet me at my baptism. I remembered her rollicking chuckle, and how she had taken time to chat with the children. I remembered all their India friends and co-laborers who would have loved to come honor her memory on this occasion. I remembered working with Cleason and Mary in Bulgaria, where they were my houseparents. I remembered her full life lived well, and regretted that the end was thus unhonored and unsung.

But I knew Mary, and I knew that while no eulogies could pay her the tributes she had earned, she would have been satisfied and amused to know that circumstances had conspired to hinder crowds from making a fuss over her.

After reminiscing by the casket, we walked out to let the next family walk in. We drove down the parking lot to where the mourning family waited to "meet" us at the exit lane. Brother Cleason and his family were lined up in their vehicles on both sides of the lane. It was a pleasant spring evening, and their doors and windows stood open so we could drive from one to the next and offer our condolences without physical contact. We were doing the best we could to respect the regulations and still remain a brotherhood, but family visitation lines via vans are simply awkward. Instead of strong, silent handshakes and tear stains on shoulders, we were forced to holler Profound Sentiments through car windows.

Still, it was good to see Cleason surrounded by family. God had answered many prayers; his three children from the

United States were all able to be present. The in-laws who didn't have Canadian passports could not cross the border, nor could any US grandchildren or great-grandchildren, but his children were there.

The next morning was Mary's funeral. Dad (presiding bishop) and Galen (slightly nervous sound tech responsible for three call-in systems) went to church. So did the other local ministry who had part.

None of the Martin family went to the church for the funeral service. By the time the ministry and the sound tech were there, only a handpicked few of the family could have legally gone. So the family decided none of them would go. They sat together in their living room and phoned in like the rest of us.

The service went well, if somewhat oddly, considering the lack of casket or mourners or congregation, and considering that the brother who led in devotions did so from a thousand kilometers (620 miles) away. The ministry read a few hymns in lieu of the usual singing.

Later that afternoon the Martin family gathered for the graveside service. That occasion was family only, except for the cemetery committee, the bishop, and his wife. Mom said that after all the years she and Dad had worked with Cleason and Mary in the ministry, she *was* going to this funeral. She went, but stayed inside the church house and watched from the window.

The rest of us were present only in spirit, but Dad narrated the proceedings for the sake of the in-laws and grandchildren and old friends calling in from around the world. "Now the pallbearers are lowering the casket. . . . Now they are returning to the parking lot so the family can come up to the graveside. . . . " The grandchildren and great-grandchildren filed past, and then returned to their vehicles so Mary's brothers and sisters could take their turn at the graveside. Finally, when it was time for the committal, the only people in the cemetery were Cleason, his children, and Dad.

I know about funerals; I've been to half a hundred, and this was certainly the strangest one I never was at. But God promised to attend where two or three gather, and that day He came to comfort ten.

Quarantine Family Challenge

Gina Martin

ON A SUNDAY evening in late March 2020, my six children and I sat with a few of my siblings by a campfire in my parents' backyard. In the past two weeks our schedules had crumbled, and we had formed new routines for Sunday services at home. *Shelter-in-place* and *social distancing* were now familiar terms.

I wasn't worried about the virus. My husband had died of brain cancer less than a year before, and I knew God's presence in difficult times. But the Pennsylvania governor was expected to enact a stay-at-home order for our county within a few days, which would increase our isolation. We would miss spending time with cousins and friends.

As the fire crackled, my siblings and I discussed the quarantine. Without church and social events, we would need activities to keep us busy. We wanted to respect the government rulings while finding ways to connect with others. For our emotional well-being, we needed goals.

I don't know who suggested the idea, but before we said good night, we had begun the first week of our Quarantine Family Challenge.

Each week one of us nine siblings chose five or six challenges and messaged them to the rest of the family. Throughout the week we reported our progress. There was no pressure, so if a particular challenge didn't work for my family, we skipped it. But knowing others were also doing the challenges motivated us to complete most of them.

Some challenges got us outdoors to search for wildflowers, watch a sunrise, sleep in a tent in the backyard, plant a tree in memory of COVID-19, and identify the North Star.

Other challenges encouraged serving others by sending a card to an elderly person or making a meal for someone. Serving others helped us get our minds off our own problems.

Thankfully, the quarantine coincided with the coming of spring, which allowed us to get outdoors for exercise. We were challenged to bike five miles and play kickball or croquet as a family. One of the highlights was when we all walked or ran a 5K and reported our times; the contested times led to another family 5K later that summer to find the true winners.

We were challenged to try new things: learn a new song, memorize a Bible verse, try a new recipe, and learn about an unfamiliar country. One week we were challenged to *upcycle*—to make something new out of something old. At our house, the result was a goat shed built out of old metal.

Some challenges lived up to that name. Writing a poem was one project that didn't go so well for most of us. The children were challenged to not argue with their siblings for a day, while the adults were challenged to turn off their phones and not use the Internet for a whole day.

Our challenges lasted nine weeks—the length of our county's stay-at-home order. At the end of that time, we had resumed Sunday-morning services and could once again gather in person with extended family and friends. Although I was glad to resume normal life, I missed those intentional challenges. They had pushed us to try new things, connected us with family, and provided a needed focus for unscheduled days. We would probably benefit from having a similar program every spring.

Research has shown that we are much more likely to meet a goal if we tell someone about it and report our progress. Whether the goal is exercising, decluttering the house, or reading a book, it is more fun when a friend is working toward the same goal so we can encourage each other.

We need the strength of each other in hard times. During the months surrounding my husband's illness and death, I felt the strength of our family and church. But I also learned that when I'm stressed, I can become critical of others and annoyed over small things. Tempers can fray and offenses mount when I need others the most. During times like a pandemic, we can bicker like bored children—or we can challenge each other to rest in the Lord and to serve others in love.

In the family of God—the Church—we must challenge one another to live for Jesus Christ until we escape the quarantine of this stricken world and go Home to stay.

Under His Wings

Hannah Myers

GOD ASKS US to trust Him—and we want to—but sometimes our faith falters. We tend to forget His omnipresence. We wonder just how wide His wingspan reaches.

On March 15, Florida Mennonite Fellowship of Colonia Florida, Paraguay, officially closed its front church doors in accordance with COVID-19 restrictions: no public services. We compromised by dividing into four groups at designated homes each Sunday.

One month into this routine, the ministers desired to hold a members' meeting. If "members only" consisted of less than half the congregation, dare we try one short meeting in our dear *capilla*?

The meeting was scheduled for an odd hour, two o'clock on a Sunday afternoon. A small collection of vans, pickups, and motorcycles crowded the yard behind the church house, the space least seen from the road.

The meeting commenced. While the bishop was speaking, a young brother felt his muted cell phone vibrating. He hit "off." Several seconds later, it vibrated again. He silenced it.

Another youth's phone vibrated. Swift strides took him outside. He quickly returned. "We've been reported! The police are on their way out!"

In a flash, the bishop wound up his words and adjourned the meeting. We fled.

Three months later, when phase four of reopening was in effect, three young girls were waiting for believer's baptism. Dare we try again?

This time we opted for private property, back a long lane. An implement shed behind a banana patch seemed ideal, except the open side of the building faced the road—visible at a distance. The solution? The farmer moved his tractor and hay equipment from the inside to the outside. Lined up just right, they covered the span seen from the road.

Another Sunday afternoon and a different odd hour. The whole congregation arrived. We sat—with bated breath—on a peculiar assortment of chairs and waited in silence.

The meeting commenced. The deacon spoke of the privilege of gathering again as a united group, of the joy of souls saved, and of rejoicing that the church on earth is growing.

Then the applicants, Cindy Cantero, Heather Myers, and Sharla Myers, stood and solemnly vowed to serve God the rest of their lives. They knelt on a piece of linoleum. Water poured over their bowed heads in the name of the Father, the Son, and the Holy Ghost and dripped onto *hallowed ground.* They arose, baptized into the church of God.

The congregation relaxed—no interference from authorities! We opened our thirsty hearts toward heaven and allowed the water of the Word to wash over our souls. The bishop preached a soul-stirring sermon, beseeching us to be true to our commitment to Christ because the devil will try his utmost to destroy faith in God. We listened in reverence.

The meeting closed. We slipped home one by one. *In peace.* "If God be for us, who can be against us?"

Rusty tin...gravel floor...undercover...

But in the *shadow* of the *Almighty.*

COVID-19 and the Morses

Kurt & Naomi Morse

ACCORDING TO MR. MORSE:

My wife and I had just settled into the administrator's apartment at the Gingerich Home for the Elderly in Farmington when COVID-19 reached New Mexico. Since the facility was without a resident administrator at the time, we had been asked to move there to serve in some hybrid combination of houseparents for the staff, advisors for the daily operations of the facility, and a stabilizing presence at the Home.

As the state began to implement laws to control the spread of COVID-19, I expected the restrictions to last for a few weeks, perhaps a month. Then life would return to normal. Not so. A new "normal" began to settle over the land, and it seemed to become heavily concentrated over the Gingerich Home.

The staff at the Gingerich Home, all nine of them, were normal Mennonite girls who enjoyed an active social life. With the restrictions the state implemented, along with the precautions put in place by the Gingerich Home board, the staff soon felt as if they had been placed in a convent in some very out-of-the-way place.

In general, the guidelines for the GH were stricter than those the state mandated. We knew that the best way to keep COVID out of the Home was to keep it away from the staff. This meant restricted lifestyles for all of us, as well as quarantines for new workers and any workers coming back from trips.

It was amazing what questions the girls could come up with in conjunction with the new restrictions. "Wouldn't it be okay if we went to...?" or "Does that mean I can't...?"

My reply was "What part of 'Stay home' don't you understand?" I began to feel like a tyrannical dictator. With time though, we all learned to live with less social life and to find satisfaction in the routine. We found it was easier for the girls to cope with this if they believed their sacrifice really *was* helping to keep the residents safe.

The residents of the Gingerich Home had an even more restricted reality than the staff. No visitors—period. Many of their family members used ingenuity to find legal ways to stay in touch, such as visiting by phone through a closed window. To some, the rules seemed almost unbearable, and they pled with us to bend them. Again, I felt like a tyrant, but I knew that starting on that course would only bring a flood of new questions.

At the onset of the pandemic, it was thought best for all the staff, including my wife and me, to refrain from shopping in town. This was a great hardship for the girls we were supervising. The board chairman, Harley Kauffman, and his wife were designated as shoppers for the Gingerich Home and staff, since they were not in direct contact with the residents. This was a huge undertaking for them, especially because many essentials were not available.

Eventually, I was allowed to do some of our own shopping, since I was not in as close contact with the residents as my wife was. My appreciation for cell phones skyrocketed as many questions surfaced during these trips. "Naomi, what brand of baking powder do you like?" Five minutes later, "They don't have the bacon that was supposed to be on sale. Should I get a different kind?" Four minutes later, "I thought cabbage was cheap. This head costs about five dollars. Should I get it anyway?" And on and on the questions went.

My dear wife remained patient, and perhaps a bit amused, despite the seven calls she received from me in one morning. The subsequent shopping trips went better, and she started to worry about me when a whole shopping trip went by without a call.

The girls were thankful when they were finally given permission to go to town once a week for necessities. My wife also got back to shopping sometimes, but she claims she got spoiled by letting me do it.

It is now August 2020, and COVID-19 has been a dominating presence in our lives these last five months. In this time, I have accepted the position of administrator of the Gingerich Home, which means my responsibilities have increased. We can reflect on things we have missed out on, such as our hoped-for trip to Switzerland this summer to visit Anabaptist historical sights. This was scrapped when no European travel was permitted. Our plans for visiting family in New York and Pennsylvania have been postponed indefinitely.

Sometimes, we feel we can relate to portions of 2 Corinthians 4:8, 9. "*We are troubled on every side*, yet not distressed." In our human weakness, we can give extra attention to the trouble we face without allowing God to ease our distresses. "*We are perplexed*, but not in despair." Perplexity is a condition we may face, but despair is not necessary if we have God. "*Persecuted*, but not forsaken." The restrictions placed on us may have caused us to feel a trifle persecuted, but God has not forsaken the staff or the residents.

The Lord has blessed our efforts. None of the staff or residents have tested positive for COVID-19. And if He should choose to allow that yet, He will give us a way through. We may feel "*cast down*," but we are "not destroyed." Not by the troubles, the perplexities, the restrictions, the missed vacations, or the shopping trips.

Oh, by the way, I actually enjoyed my shopping experiences.

—Kurt P. Morse

ACCORDING TO MRS. MORSE:

When the shopping mania first hit our town, we were determined not to become part of it. Surely this was a lot of hype over nothing. We entertained ourselves with discussions of how to manufacture our own paper products and hand sanitizer. But when weeks went by, and there really were no replacements in sight for the ever-decreasing paper products, we started feeling something akin to fear in the pits of our stomachs.

What *would* we do with fourteen seniors in a house with no paper products? Nor Clorox? Nor sanitizer? Worse yet—what *would* happen if this virus swept through our Home? And how *will* we keep it out? This was only the beginning of what seemed like at least a million questions we asked ourselves and each other in the next few months.

Day and night, our brains weighed the questions: What is safe and what is sensible? Our vulnerable residents were at our mercy. At first, we felt like heroes gathering them all into a safe cave while a fire passed by. But after a month and then two and three and more—we didn't feel like heroes anymore. We just felt like people stuck in the same cave with the same people day after day with no escape in view. Should we take a few risks and bring some normalcy to everyone's life?

I overheard two residents conversing at the breakfast table. "Well, nobody's caught the virus yet," said Martha[8] in an attempt at being cheerful.

"Oh, we won't," returned Dottie, "because we don't go anywhere, and these girls don't go anywhere, and nobody comes in. So, we won't have a chance of catching it. We can be very thankful for that."

"Well, I don't know," said Martha. "I figure if I get sick, then I just get sick." The confinement was depressing for her. Was it worth taking their "life" away to "save their lives"? But most of that question was already answered by the state. Keeping up with changing state regulations, and the constant reporting required, was an overwhelming job that supervisor Elisabeth Miller shouldered bravely.

The term "safe" became a relative term for the staff. Our winter had already been traumatic. In January, our friend Sasha Krause had been abducted from our church house (or grounds) and later found murdered. The girls, who had for many years freely walked to and from work, day or night, often right through the church grounds, were instructed to "be safe and don't go alone."

Now two months later, "be safe" meant staying away from people. Perplexing, to say the least. Giving direction on these questions fell heavily on my husband, Kurt, and on the board chairman, Harley Kauffman. Many hours of discussion and phone calls passed between them. Sometimes when the girls asked Kurt a question, he would say, "I don't know; ask Harley."

"Harley said to ask you!" they would reply.

Once Harley told the girls he had "no more answers until next week."

What other sides of us have been brought out by this virus? In these days, what feel like selfish actions are actually for the cause of unselfishness. Small children don't understand that I stay away from them because of my responsibility to protect the elderly. Adults can understand better, but when new workers come, and we need to make them hole up in some room until they've proven themselves "safe." It feels so un-Christian to do this to them. They came to help us, and we treat them like criminals. I hope we won't forget what hospitality is supposed to look like. But then I go back to the reality: if I were the one to bring COVID-19 into our Home, everyone would suffer. And if anyone would get sick and die, I would have a hard time forgiving myself. That thought has often given me the persistence to keep up the required unselfish "selfishness."

We've heard that masks cover people's smiles. However, one morning after a new worker arrived, I overheard one resident say to her neighbor, "Did you see what a pretty smile she has?" The new worker had been wearing a mask all morning, so it wasn't her mouth our resident saw. So, smile behind your mask. It shows.

What have we learned through the pandemic pandemonium? Perhaps we'll know better later. One thing I learned is that we can live on less social life and shopping. I hope I'm learning what God wants me to. We certainly have had to call on Him many times for wisdom. The song "He Giveth More Grace" uses this phrase, "When we reach the end of our hoarded resources, our Father's full giving has only begun."[9] That has been so true!

The paper products and hand sanitizer never completely ran out, and Harley's supply of answers always got replenished before the next week. And none of our residents died of boredom. Day after day, our dedicated staff members come back to work with enough grace to do their duties and. And we know God will give enough grace for every tomorrow, as well.

—Naomi Morse

---

9   Annie Johnson Flint, "He Giveth More Grace"

Revival in a Rocking Boat

Darletta F. Martin

A HURRICANE OF questions swirled around our revival meetings.

Should we have them or should we not? The law finally allowed us to hold services again after nine stay-at-home Sundays. Would it be pushing the limits to also hold a week of revivals in the middle of June?

Communion, Good Friday, Easter, and Ascension Day meetings had been canceled. What if we planned for revivals, only to be restricted at the last minute from having them?

Did all the members agree that we should have meetings? No. Because one couple in our congregation had tested positive for COVID-19, some members did not feel comfortable attending church. Others declared that Pondsville has held a week of revivals every summer for more than sixty years, and COVID was not a good reason to skip it.

Was the evangelist willing to come? Yes. Someone in his own congregation had tested positive, so the risk wasn't any greater in our community. He was ready to drive an hour each evening to inspire us with God's Word.

Would revival meetings be pleasant in these circumstances? Usually, the hot weather and huge crowds make our small church house stuffy and sticky. This year the weather was moderate. The crowd would be small since visitors were asked to listen on the conference line instead of attending in person. But those of us who enjoy socializing knew we would miss the fellowship.

Since no government regulations deterred them, the ministry announced their plans to go ahead with the scheduled meetings.

Then a tsunami struck. On the Thursday evening before the week of meetings began, our fifteen-year-old friend Argyl suffered severe burns from a propane burner when attempting to dry the plaster in a cistern. Although Argyl's family is part of another congregation, he was the beloved grandson, nephew, cousin, friend, and coworker of many in our congregation. He was life-flighted to a burn center in Washington, DC, where his parents sent reports from his bedside for the next four days.

What a shock! How could we steady the boat for our friends and family? While our son Dalen had been separated from most of his classmates since March, he and Argyl had been spending at least two days a week together, working at Keith's Calf Barn. Their jolly times had spilled over into our household, adding laughter to meals and spice to spare moments.

Could we hold revivals in this storm? No one canceled the meetings, so the evangelist came on Sunday evening. Some of us scattered across the church auditorium while others chose to listen from home. A small group met again on Monday evening.

On Tuesday morning, Argyl's family sent out word that his organs were shutting down. For the first time, his siblings were allowed to gather around his bed. They waited there until the angels carried him Home in the afternoon.

How could we calmly ride out revival meetings in such a tempest? Our local minister was Argyl's uncle. We didn't expect their family to come, nor Argyl's grandmother and other relatives.

No one called off the service, so we opened the church building according to schedule. We sat down wearily with a few others and tearfully sang "Safe in the Arms of Jesus."

I doubted whether revival was possible that night.

Our evangelist, Kevin Ebersole, was not a stranger to grief. When he was twenty-one, two of his brothers had died from meningitis. He spoke openly of our loss and expressed his sympathy. Then he told us that after he received word of Argyl's death, he'd had one hour in which to exchange the sermon he had planned for the evening with one more appropriate for the circumstances. He titled it "The Reason for Storms."

He reminded us of Jesus's words, "Be of good cheer; it is I; be not afraid." The disciples were doing what Jesus had instructed them to do, so why did they need to experience a storm?

God sends storms either to correct us or to perfect us. He wants us to understand who Jesus is. When the disciples could not see Jesus, He was on the mountain praying for them. Satan wants to trick us into thinking Jesus has deserted us.

THE LIVING OF THESE DAYS

Jesus allowed Peter to walk on the water to show us that faith can conquer fear. Faith can move us forward to Jesus if we keep our focus on Him. When Jesus enters our boat, we are safer in the storm than out of it.

Brother Kevin concluded his message by reminding us that storms don't last forever. When tranquility comes, we praise God for His goodness and wonder why we feared the storm.

Calmness settled over our small group of disciples as we felt Jesus's presence in our rocking boat. The same God Who allowed the surges had sent us revival before we drowned. He would strengthen our faith to tread the waters of sorrow in the following days.

The Master's Symphony

Deborah Coblentz

OUR LOFTY ASPIRATIONS for the smooth-flowing symphony
of this term
      fractured
            before the end of the opening score.
   The Conductor beat a rest—fermata—
      until the silence rang.

When we resumed, He reassigned our parts.
I had been a soprano, but now I sing the descant.
      The alto was replaced.
And now—we sing along together, learning to harmonize,
      faltering at unfamiliar words and music.

> But we sing, with our eyes on the Conductor,
>   lest there should be discordant notes.
> For He is the Maestro and—in the end—
>   His song will be glorious.

After I began teaching in Florida Colony five years ago, I concluded that school terms in Paraguay are less predictable than their North American counterparts. No matter how well I think I've prepared myself for the unexpected, God's arrangements still stretch my capacity.

Absences punctuated our 2019 term. One first grader's family returned from a trip to Peru several days after classes began. Another student left in May. In June, the tragic death of co-teacher Carolina's brother-in-law spurred her return to Honduras for two weeks. And when three Myers families simultaneously spent time States-side for the first time in years, even the cushioning two weeks of midterm vacation did not completely absorb the bumps of students working ahead and catching up to their classmates afterward.

After a year like that, our hopes swelled for a *normal* term in 2020—at least, more nearly normal. Classes commenced on February 20. But we were only sixteen days into establishing routine when several confirmed coronavirus cases in Paraguay prompted the government-issued mandate: no school for two weeks.

Two weeks passed. The quarantine was extended . . . two more weeks . . . and two more. Realizing it might be months before school resumed, our upper-grade teacher, Carolyn Yoder, returned to the United States on a repatriation flight. Carolina

Sanchez and I stayed, doing whatever our hands found to do. And we exercised sitting still, until . . . Until when?

In mid-May, after eight weeks of no school, we began circuit-teaching, dropping off assignments at the beginning of the week and collecting them each Friday. Although it was better than nothing, it seemed a far cry from genuine classroom learning.

June rolled in. I had just prepared assignments for the sixth week of homeschool when the school board proposed resuming classes at separate locations. Since the border was still closed, would Carolina and I consent to adding Carolyn's students to our own?

Too overjoyed at the prospect of teaching again to feel overwhelmed by the added responsibility of two more grades and five more students, I consented in a heartbeat. Heather Myers agreed to be my helper. Three action-packed days later, classes resumed. Heather and I, with our thirteen students, were snugly tucked into a church family's guest house. Carolina's class met in a basement on the neighboring farm.

Initially, we had hoped this would be a temporary arrangement. But the weeks roll by with no end to quarantine restrictions in sight, and we have adapted to this strange new normal. No visiting brethren for devotions, no hot lunches, but a joint recess with Carolina's class each Friday!

Usually, our school term ends in October; this term—because of the three-month intermission—we hope to finish in December. But God is the composer of this school term, and we await His direction, giving thanks for the privilege of educating our children.

We've adjusted our expectations, yes, and we even harmonize, joyfully singing the Master's symphony.

Through Heaven's Gates

Sara Nolt

She wasn't my grandma until I married John. But once our vows were sealed, Verna Fox so fully adopted me into the family that I felt as though I had always belonged to her. I received her kiss on my cheek and heard her quavering voice speak the Blessing of Aaron over me: "'The Lord *bless* you and keep you. The Lord make His face *shine* upon you...and give you *peace.*'"

Grandma spoke the passage with such depth and conviction that the verses were not empty recitations. Grandma loved the Lord and talked to Him often about her family, something that comforted me when John and I prepared to move to Ghana.

One evening, when our preparations for traveling were complete, we stopped by Grandma's house to say goodbye. The house hadn't changed in the ten years of our marriage. Our children now played at Grandma's feet with the same toys John had played with when he was a boy.

Grandma herself was the same. When I hugged her goodbye, surprisingly strong hands gripped my shoulders. With depth and purpose, she spoke the Blessing of Aaron over our family and promised to pray for us.

I hoped to see her when we returned. She was in excellent health, but we knew that could change rapidly in a ninety-five-year-old lady.

Indeed, Grandma's health declined while we were in Ghana. We received a message that Grandma was in the hospital. At one point, she grew so weak, so limp, that the nurses thought they had lost her. "Are you still with us, Verna?"

Grandma awoke at the sound of their voices. When she was able to speak, Grandma told the family, "I saw the beautiful gates of heaven and was walking toward them. But then someone called my name."

Sweet Grandma! She returned to a hospital bed and an ailing body—a disappointment for someone who was homesick for heaven.

Grandma rallied and moved into Fairmount Homes, an assisted-living facility. John and I visited her there when we returned from Ghana. By now she was ninety-eight, nearly blind, nearly deaf, but she still exuded the sweetness, faith, and strength I so admired.

Enter COVID-19. To protect the elderly, visitors were not allowed in nursing homes. Grandma's steady flow of family and friends abruptly stopped. Volunteers were also kept away. Fairmount's nurses and staff are stellar caregivers, so we knew Grandma was in capable hands. But even the best nurses are mortal and limited. They couldn't sit and chat like family, nor give relaxed, focused attention as volunteers could.

Grandma's health deteriorated quickly. Within weeks of the new restrictions, she developed a tickle in her throat. She said, "It feels like I might be getting a cold."

With a deadly virus running rampant and with so many vulnerable people in their care, the staff couldn't risk exposing other residents to a cold. They quarantined Grandma in her room. Nurses occasionally dropped by to check on her or to bring meals, but mostly, Grandma sat alone.

The loneliness was hard to handle, but greater than a lost social life was the loss of the routines that had defined her day. She couldn't mark the passing of time by going to devotions, the activity room, or the dining hall. Barren hours stretched endlessly before her.

Being nearly blind complicated the new restrictions. Grandma could still see slivers of light, but she couldn't identify its source. Was it sunshine or the her room's nighttime light? She could not tell. Day and night melted into a long, uncomfortable existence.

That tickle in Grandma's throat developed into a nasty cough, which the doctor diagnosed as the final stages of heart disease. Her breathing became labored. Death was on its way. Unable to get enough oxygen when lying down, Grandma stayed in her recliner.

Grandma didn't complain, but when my mother-in-law called Grandma one morning and said, "Hello, Mom," she heard relief in Grandma's response—relief that tore at all our hearts.

"Is it really morning?" Grandma replied. "Oh, I'm so glad to know the sun is shining outside."

Another long night was over.

Fairmount's remarkable nurses did what they could to be Grandma's friend, but with their heavy workload, they couldn't sit with her by the hour, which was what Grandma really needed. The woman who had nurtured a dozen children of her own and cared for ten foster babies now suffered with no one to return the favor.

Sometimes longing crept into her voice. She didn't want to die alone. Nobody wanted her to. Grandma's children called the home, trying to find some way to be with Grandma.

"Can just one person wear full protective gear and come sit with her?" they asked.

The nursing home administrator was apologetic, but unrelenting. "I'm so sorry. We cannot allow it."

With state restrictions tying their hands, the best Fairmount could do for the family was to let some of them stand outside Grandma's bedroom window and sing. The window had to remain shut, and Grandma's vision was too impaired for her to see outside. Still, it comforted her to know that her children were so close.

But they weren't close enough.

I hated the idea of our sweet grandma sitting by herself in a dark, quiet world, struggling to breathe. I asked my mother-in-law, "Why don't you take Grandma to someone's house? Then family could be with her all the time."

The more the family considered the idea, the more they thought it was possible. But it wasn't as easy as picking her up and whisking her away. They needed to secure oxygen, for by now Grandma was on oxygen full-time. They needed an ambulance as transportation and hospice to come after she was settled. And she needed to be released from Fairmount.

But that couldn't happen too soon; Grandma was rapidly declining. She spent one night in a coma and was considered actively dying. Thankfully, the state permits immediate family to sit with dying patients. When Grandma regained consciousness, two family members—the maximum allowed—were by her side. Other children gratefully congregated in a reception room, waiting their turns and singing. Those sitting with Grandma turned on a speakerphone so she could hear the songs.

"Sing 'I Need No Mansion Here Below' for Mom," one daughter told the group.

Grandma thought Auntie had spoken to her, so she began to sing. But instead of with the quavering, gasping voice that could only manage a word or two at a time, Grandma sang with the strength of her youth, her voice unwavering and clear. She sang the entire song without getting winded. To her daughters sitting with her, Grandma's song was heaven's gift.

Due to the severity of Grandma's condition, arrangements were expedited. It felt like a celebration to us all when we knew Grandma was at her daughter's house. At last, the siblings gathered around their mother, told her goodbye, and gave her all their pent-up love and care. Comforted, Grandma slipped inside heaven's gates less than thirty hours after her release from Fairmount. She was ninety-nine years, nine months, and twenty days old.

COVID restrictions complicated funeral plans; we were informed that only ten people could attend a graveside service.

Ten people. Grandma had ten surviving children. The rest of the family—spouses, 57 grandchildren, 218 great-grandchildren, and 67 great-great-grandchildren—could not attend.

The funeral home arranged for the graveside service to be live-streamed, so from my kitchen table, I saw the hearse arrive at the site and watched the funeral director open the back door. I teared up as eight siblings, my mother-in-law included, stepped forward. When there are only ten attendees, mourners double as pallbearers. The viewing was brief but tender. Just a few people to whisper goodbye and speak words of encouragement and comfort to each other. Then, standing in front of their mother's casket, they sang songs of hope and heaven. An ordained son preached a message for a live-streamed audience. Other siblings shared poems and memories. They prayed. They sang. Together, they lowered their mother's body to its resting place.

For Grandma, death was a release from a tired body and a restricted life in a COVID-infested world. But at the time of this writing, the virus continues to narrow the margins of living for many senior citizens. Caregivers are doing their best to protect the vulnerable by building a wall between them and a deadly virus. Activities are canceled. Visitors are limited. Loneliness is their companion.

When restrictions lift—as they surely will someday—I want to remember the elderly. I want to surround them with care and love until they, too, can step peacefully through heaven's gates.

The Mexican Odyssey

Kervin Martin

ON THE EVENING of July 28, 2020, an ambulance slowed as it approached a farm lane in northern Ohio. There were no flashing lights and no siren. It made its way up the driveway and parked beside the house. The throaty rumble of the engine died, and all was still.

Inside the house, the Fox family was just finishing their supper. The arrival of an ambulance on their farm was definitely unusual, but they had been expecting it. Victor Fox rose from his place at the table and greeted the driver at the door. I stepped in. "Good evening! Good to see you again, Victor."

"Yeah, are you ready for a long trip?"

"I guess so."

Both Victor and I are twenty-five, and we have been on long trips before. This trip, however, was going to be different from any we had ever taken before and probably would ever take again. The reason for the trip was simple. Victor's wedding had been scheduled for four days ago, yet he was still some 1,800 miles from his bride, who was in Honduras. The logistics behind choosing an ambulance to make the trip were more complex.

A virus had spread across the globe, causing many countries to close their borders to land, sea, and air travel. Victor had not even seen his girlfriend, Karolina, for more than five months. To fix that issue, he was now on the verge of trying the unthinkable, driving an ambulance three thousand miles across three international borders to Honduras. The ambulance would be a donation to the health department of Honduras, so the trip fell under the category of humanitarian aid. Victor had asked me to go with him on this adventure. I had taught school in Colombia, South America, for two years, so I was familiar with the culture and language we would encounter along the way.

The next morning, we were on our way south. I estimated we could get to Honduras in a week or two. We reached the Mexican border on the second day of our travels, and here we met the first speed bump in our journey. Several days before reaching Mexico, I had sent our paperwork to an agent at the Mexican border so he would have the seventy-two hours normally required to process a vehicle that would permanently leave the country. When we got to the office, we found that some of the paperwork had not gone through, but the agents assured us all would be ready in three days. We had no choice but to wait.

We enjoyed a trip to the ocean, some fishing, and many delicious meals at Mexican restaurants. On the third day, we arrived at the agency office with high hopes, but after we had waited for seven hours, they informed us that our paperwork could not be processed. I spent the rest of the day making phone calls to various contacts, trying to figure out what could be done next.

Late in the evening, I got a message from a local broker with whom I had been in contact. I explained the situation, and the broker responded that we should not worry, he was sure he could help. The next day, he took us to another agency, which was very nice to work with, and gave us high hopes that they could process our papers. They even gave the option of providing a custodian to help us travel to Guatemala.

It took another three days for this agency to process the paperwork, but on August 6, we successfully crossed into Mexico, after waiting at the border for a full week. Unfortunately, the custodian who was going with us had plans to help another vehicle through the border before he could go with us. This other vehicle finally came through a day later. After eight days of waiting, both of us were ready to travel.

In two days, we were at the Guatemala border. We hoped we could cross soon. We soon realized, however, that connecting with all the right agents and officials was not going to be easy. Mexico was ready to let us through, but Guatemala was not interested in letting us in until they knew for sure that Honduras would let us through their border. I made more calls and was told that the department of health in Honduras would settle the issue with Guatemala in a few days.

Victor and I crossed into Guatemala on foot and visited friends who lived near the border. After fifteen days on the road, spending time with trustworthy people of like faith was refreshing.

On August 18, Victor heard that Honduras was beginning international flights again. Meanwhile, our contacts who were trying to help us get the ambulance into Guatemala were not making much headway. The fact that we were doing humanitarian aid helped, but the process was still slow. The question was not if we could get through, but when. We would also need to have a Guatemalan drive the ambulance through the country for us, so we decided that maybe returning to the United States would be our best option. Victor and the ambulance would still both get to Honduras, though probably at different times.

We said goodbye to our friends in Guatemala and checked tickets to return to the States. By early afternoon, Victor and I were back in Mexico and in a taxi bound for a hotel near the Tapachula airport. I had already booked my flight for the next day and was looking over my itinerary when our taxi was pulled over by armed officers.

The taxi doors opened, and one of the officers peered into the back. Spotting two foreigners, he motioned us out of the vehicle. He checked our passports and also looked over the visa card we had gotten upon entering the country. The visas we had were good for seven days, which was actually a mistake, since we had asked and paid for 180 days.

We had already learned that the border official who gave us the card had taken advantage of us, giving us seven free days and keeping our money for himself. We had tried to get new visas on the day before they expired, but immigration officials had told us not to worry. We didn't need new visas, but would have to pay a fee whenever we left Mexico. I explained this to the officer detaining us, but he said no, this was a problem and needed to be fixed. He explained he would take us to a place that would help us with our visas. It sounded simple enough, so we paid the taxi driver, and he drove off.

The officers ushered us into the back of a waiting security van, and we drove for about ten minutes. I thought it a little strange that the immigration officials in the office had said we were fine, and now these men, who were also immigration officials, were saying we had a problem. I wasn't worried, however. I figured we could straighten everything out in short order and be back at our hotel for the night.

When we arrived at our destination, I began to wonder just a bit. Armed guards opened two large gates and let our van into a compound. We stopped at a large building and were ordered into a simple room with only concrete benches to sit on. At one end of the room was a desk, cluttered with miscellaneous paper junk. Seven officials examined what valuables we had with us.

We were told to remove our shoelaces because "they are not permitted in this building." We also had to hand over all our electronics and all our money. I was trying to figure out what this all had to do with talking to an immigration official and getting a new visa. Our clothing was then separated from the rest of our luggage and the remaining contents put in plastic bags "to be put in a safe until we leave."

Leaving all our things in the hands of the officials, we were taken to an office, where an immigration officer named Juan gave us some forms to fill out. As he answered my questions as to what was happening, I realized we were being held as illegal immigrants. This was an INM (National Institute of Immigration) prison known as Siglo XXI, the largest in the country, and we were the newest inmates. I explained our situation, and he seemed to understand but added that he was obligated by law to keep us until the US embassy moved on our behalf. I asked if we could at least call our families to let them know what had happened, and they kindly let both of us make short calls.

We were then walked back to the main part of the prison and assured that usually the US embassy acts quickly, often within twenty-four hours. As we were escorted through several heavy metal doors, I took in the sights, sounds, and smells of our new home. The men's section of the complex consisted of halls of cells holding up to fifty men each, a shower room, and a dining area. An outdoor courtyard was surrounded by a steel fence, then a concrete wall topped by rolls of barbed wire. A guard tower stood on top of the wall that separated the men's and women's courtyards.

Around seven hundred men from over ten countries lounged, dozed, or simply sauntered aimlessly about. The walls resounded with a continuous hum of chattering, whooping, and jeering. The slowly circulating air inside seemed to gain putrid potential as it wafted from cell to cell. Stories of Christians imprisoned for their faith flashed through my mind as I took it all in. *So maybe this is a taste of what it's like*, I thought.

At this point, I felt just as much intrigue as apprehension. I had always been interested in visiting a pen of this nature, though it had definitely not been on my list for that day. I breathed a prayer that God would give us the strength for whatever this adventure might bring. I also prayed that God would help me to surrender myself to whatever His purpose was for me here.

Guards took us to a private cell and asked if we preferred that, or if we would rather sleep with the others. I felt a bit guilty but said a private cell would be great. So, we found ourselves in cell DE-4, having no clue how long we would be in this thirteen-by-eight-foot room. There was a concrete shelf that served as a bed frame for one of us, a rusty tap and sink, and a commode that sat quite exposed in the corner. We were each given a thin mattress, a light blanket, and a scanty pack of toiletry items. With that, the guards left us to ourselves.

There we sat, with nothing but the clothes on our backs and our Bibles. I had asked a guard if we could please take our Bibles with us, and he agreed. We made ourselves as comfortable as we could, and the guards soon came around to lock our cells for the night. We read our Bibles for some time, prayed, and somehow fell into a light sleep, the bulbs of the prison shining down on us the whole night.

Around seven o'clock the next morning, the guards unlocked our cell, and we followed a herd of men to the courtyard outside, joining the few hundred men already there. Heads turned as two Americans came out of the compound. We explained, first to one group, then to another, who we were and why we were there.

It became apparent that these were just regular men, not criminals. Though everyone was supposedly in Mexico illegally, some had about the same story as we did. There were even a few other Americans there. We quickly made friends with some fellows from Colombia, and they explained how the place operated.

At mealtimes, we made a line along the outside wall of the building before we were let into the dining area. The line in the dining area wound around the room till it got to the kitchen window where we got our food. Each morning, we were given a slip of paper divided into three sections: breakfast, lunch, and supper. To get our food tray, we would need to hand in our tickets at the kitchen window. Each meal was about the same: five to seven corn tortillas, beans, and sometimes rice, stew, or eggs with hot dog pieces to go along. Sometimes, we got an orange or pack of crackers, too. If we were closer to the end of the line, the food was fairly cold. It was the first I ever attempted to eat twenty corn tortillas a day, but I quickly got used to it.

The best time to get a shower was usually after breakfast. Simplicity seemed to be the main focus of the shower room design. It was just a long hall full of shower stalls. There were no doors to the stalls, and the privacy walls between showers were only about five feet high. Very simple and . . . well . . . inadequate. During the day, about the only things people did were play soccer and do laundry. There were four washboards outside that we were allowed to use. The soccer goals we used as wash lines.

At the end of the day, Juan Carlos came over from the compound's main office to check on us. He had been the most friendly and helpful official we had met so far, and we begged him to let us each make a call home. We called, and found that while our parents wanted to help, there didn't seem to be much they could do for us. We went back to our cells and endured another restless night.

The next day we waited for Juan Carlos to visit, but he never showed up. It was hard to endure each day when we had no idea what was happening to get us out.

Close to the kitchen was an office with various immigration officials. I tried to ask them if there was any news of our situation, but soon found they were of no help at all. They would first explain that no, they didn't know anything, and the only thing we could do was wait. The only way to make phone calls was by getting in line with about sixty other people who also wanted to make calls. Only about ten made it through a day, and calls were restricted to two minutes each.

Five days passed with no news. We decided to make ourselves at home. We spent most of the days outdoors, visiting with everyone.

There were many men there I will never forget. One was Yefrey from Honduras. He was only about twenty-two, but he was the most inspirational person I met there. With a constant smile on his face, he read his Bible and preached to whoever was around. We sometimes sang our favorite songs together like "Por amor" ("For Love"), "En la viña del Señor" ("In the Vineyard of the Lord"), and "Yo jamás volveré" ("I Will Never Turn Back").

One evening, while we were having a Bible study in our cell, another friend popped in to listen. He was followed by a few more, and soon the doorway was full. Faces peered in from the long, narrow windows cut into the cell wall. I turned it over to Yefrey, and he began to preach about God's love for us, the plan He has for each one of us, and the kind of commitment we need to have for Him.

Yefrey encouraged me that God has a work for us to do no matter where we are. He believed that God sent him here to preach and lead others to Christ. That lesson, taught in these circumstances, affected me in a new way.

On Monday evening, August 24, I asked again if I could please speak to Juan Carlos from the main office. This time a kind INM official actually went to check for us. He returned without Juan Carlos, but at least had some info. The main boss told me we were going to leave the next day. I didn't believe it. The seven other officers in the room all looked at me like I was a few bricks short. "He just said you're going home tomorrow! What's wrong with you?"

There had been so many promises and hopes destroyed already. How was I supposed to know what the truth was when all the prisoners could watch these "professional officers" do nothing but sit around and play video games on their phones all day? I begged to call my dad, and surprisingly, they let me. It was the fourth call I had been able to make in our whole time there. He said he had just received our itinerary, and we were actually leaving. Praise the Lord!

The next afternoon we were ready to leave at four o'clock. By this time, many of the fellows had figured out we were leaving. When our names were called, everyone put up a racket of whistling and cheering. There were many high fives and handshakes as we made our way out. I was almost sad to leave, not because we were leaving a special place, but because many people there had become special to us.

Our first step upon leaving was getting our belongings back. A few small items of mine had been confiscated, but Victor had it worse; his entire supply of contacts, worth around $200, had been taken. We were transported to the Tapachula airport in a security van and escorted by police. There, we found out that because of extra security in Mexico City, each of us could only take ten kilograms (twenty-two pounds) of luggage. Victor had a lot of clothes along and had to leave a suitcase full behind.

An immigration official escorted us to Mexico City and saw us to our plane, which was headed to the States. We made it to Cleveland, Ohio, the evening of August 26, about a month after our odyssey began. The trip turned out to be different than we had anticipated, but we believe that God was at work, accomplishing more for His glory than we had dreamed.

Victor immediately started making plans to fly to Honduras. He got his COVID test done on September 3, and on September 5, he stepped on a plane bound for Honduras. By that afternoon, he was reunited with Karolina, after six months and four days of separation.

Over the next month, they went through more setbacks as they tried to get their paperwork done for their wedding. Offices were closed due to COVID, and as is common in Central America, when they did open, they didn't seem to be in a rush to get their work done. Victor said, "It seems like everything that could go wrong has gone wrong!" However, the couple was finally able to get married on October 16, eighty-four days later than they had originally planned.

God is always faithful. Though the path we tread often takes us through unexpected experiences, we have a Father we can trust—a Father Who works all things together for good.

One Night in Maine

Judi Zimmerman

THE NIGHT STARTED out as a normal night should. The sun took its time gathering all the stray rays of light and tucking them into their beds behind the horizon before darkness took over. All the little critters quieted, as well as most sane human beings. But we had to pitch our tent and put out the little fire we had built to cook our supper before climbing into the coziness of our reliable sleeping bag. Maine nights can get a little chilly, but we honeymooners had enough warmth in our hearts we didn't mind. Being in the great outdoors with the love of my life by my side was a powerful combination. In a few minutes I was asleep.

For a little while, that is. I jolted awake when my husband bolted upright and grappled with the zipper on the tent door. *Probably he heard a coon or something*, I thought from my blissful just-been-asleep state. He peered out into the darkness for a few seconds, jerked his head back inside, and whispered in a tense voice edged with fear, "Are you *sure* you're okay with sleeping here tonight?"

Warning bells reverberated in my head and goose bumps popped out all over my skin. *He's actually scared!* Whatever could have put that frightened urgency in his voice? Barely waiting for an answer, he said, "Let's throw everything in the car and leave *now*! Don't bother folding anything. Just stuff it in."

Almost two weeks prior, we had said our vows on my parents' front lawn in Kentucky. Now we were meandering along the east coast, stopping whenever the scenery called or an ice cream or lobster craving hit. The only trouble was there were half a million more attractions than we had the time to do justice to.

My husband and I are both avid lovers of practically anything outdoors, be it hiking, camping, hunting—you name it. So, it seemed only sensible to work as much of it as we could into our honeymoon, and Maine in June was the ideal place to let our adventurous side reign. We were aware of some COVID-19 restrictions, but while we were making our plans, we had thoroughly read up on Maine's current status. It didn't seem as if much would interfere, so we had headed north.

In searching for lodging, we discovered Hipcamp, the campers' version of Airbnb. Landowners clear a space in their woods or fields or down on the beach and advertise their campsite online. We were impressed the first few times with clean, secluded campsites and super-gracious hosts.

Then we booked a site called "Not for the faint of heart." Well, a lack of commodities was no problem for us—what's camping if you have every creature comfort? The hostess said she could give someone work as payment for a campsite, but we were not interested in pursuing that option. There were no reviews about the place, but maybe it was a new one. The directions to the place were slightly peculiar, but who of us doesn't have peculiarities?

We arrived early enough that we could choose a site, set up camp, cook a little supper, and retire early. At first appearances, there was no building on the place that could have been imagined livable. Items of every description graced the lawn—or the weed patch that should've been the lawn. The prominent feature on the place, an ancient farmhouse, looked as if it had lived its life and beyond. Most of the windows served no purpose as windows, since the heaps of stuff piled up inside would have deterred even the most determined ray of sunshine. A child of about twelve years of age and uncertain gender was playing under the low branches of a tree. An older woman walked out to welcome us and exclaimed over our New Mexico license plate, pointing it out to her "grandson" *(Oh, it's a boy?)* who had been "asking about New Mexico just today!"

"You may go on back and see where you wanna set up," our hostess offered, motioning to the woods beyond yet more junk languishing in the lawn that should've been. "The best spot is right behind the graveyard."

We found a path back to the woods and began our search. It turned out that behind the graveyard was the *only* place in the woods that was almost level enough to stake our tent. My husband asked numerous times if I was sure I was okay with staying. Well, I admit I wouldn't have thought of staying at a place this creepy by myself, but with my mighty prince beside me, I wasn't fazed.

By the time we had eaten and put the fire out, we were both tired enough from acting the tourist that the sleeping bag was a welcome option. I was asleep in no time at all, but unknown to me, my husband was battling fears, and praying. He asked the Lord for protection and a relaxing night and to take away his fears. Having done this, he drifted off to sleep only to jerk awake for seemingly no reason. With an uneasy, goose-bumpy feeling, he bolted out of bed and peered into the night for some sign of why he was feeling this way. Getting no answer, it seemed our only option was leaving this place *now*.

Gripped by a nameless fear, we worked swiftly and silently to pile everything into the car. Feeble yellow light glowed from two windows of the decrepit house when we passed. The digital clock on the dash of the car read 9:30 as we pulled out the driveway, and when we turned onto the road, I realized I had been holding my breath.

In a few minutes we saw the lights of the town we had left a few hours earlier. We spied a structure in the distance that looked as if it might be a hotel, so we navigated the back streets until we got closer and discovered it was a college.

We parked beside the road and employed the GPS and the Maine atlas. According to the GPS, the closest hotel with a name we recognized was about thirty minutes away. It was either drive a while or sleep in the car, which of course neither of us was keen on doing. So, we started calling hotels. Every sleepy receptionist asked the same question, "Are you in Maine on essential business?" and every one of them was sympathetic, but not enough to risk her job. "I'm really sorry, but we can't give you lodging if you are not an essential worker." We'd never encountered this dilemma before, since we'd been camping, and the campgrounds were gracious enough not to notice our out-of-state license plate.

All right, now to find a parking lot where we could be out of the way and just curl up on the seats (which couldn't lean back because the car was too full) and try to catch a few winks. Of course, the closest Walmart or any such store with a spacious parking lot was also thirty minutes away. So, we opted for a gas station. What the customers didn't realize was that it was time to be quiet and let the others at this posh hotel get some rest, so numberless times I jerked wide awake when someone hollered at a friend or cracked a hilarious joke.

The night eventually ended, and we did get some sleep. I feel I got the better end of the deal because I am considerably shorter than my husband, who had difficulty finding room for his long legs.

The following day called for a few more stops to sleep in the car—times when we were simply too exhausted to enjoy the beauties of Maine. Also included in our plans that day were reading reviews before booking a camping site and getting out of Maine as soon as possible.

Of course, we now look back and laugh at our fears, which were very likely ungrounded, but at the time we were not interested in convincing ourselves that everything was okay. Also, we would highly recommend Maine as a great place to visit, but only *after* COVID-19 is out of the picture. In fact, we were so impressed, we agreed to return for our fiftieth-anniversary trip.

From a Seven-Year Shut-In

Rhoda H. Mazelin

"HUMANS WEREN'T MADE to not go away!" Sharon declared.

True. My lips smiled in polite agreement. Humans were made to socialize, to fellowship, to mingle. God created Eve so Adam would not be alone.

Despite my outward agreement, I cringed. This year marked number seven of my being homebound. Why couldn't my friends accept a stay-at-home law? They wouldn't be shut in for half the time I had been.

Although the lives of the healthy people were majorly impacted by the shutdown (that is, if they obeyed the orders), mine wasn't. Not much at all, in fact. The biggest change was that there was more family time on Sunday, and I loved that.

Other chronically ill people also enjoyed the new normal. Lora no longer felt different; her healthy friends were also at home, reading and writing and napping. Darla felt guilty to admit it, but it was a relief not to drag her weary body out of bed in time to attend church services. Mary Ella gained strength because she no longer forced herself to go away.

Not every ill person liked the stay-at-home law. Rosetta's weakness made the extra commotion hard to tolerate. Many could not see doctors or get the treatment they depended on. Judith's health slid backward. Amy desperately needed rehydration fluids, but her condition made it riskier to go to the hospital than to endure a health crisis at home. Julee did go to the hospital, but she had to stay there alone.

Elaine was able to continue treatments at the Lyme disease clinic a thousand miles from home, but like the nurses and fellow patients, she wore a mask. She witnessed sweet staff members and sufferers being turned into short-tempered strangers due to hot masks and fear.

Fear. Thousands felt it. With rundown bodies and weak brains, the ill were especially susceptible. Susanna had reason to fear—with a compromised immune system and lung damage, she was a high-risk person.

But not all panicked. Elaine didn't. I didn't. I *was* concerned, however, because I had a severe case of mast cell activation (allergy-like reactions to almost everything), and I couldn't have done COVID-19 treatment without going heavy on Benadryl. My diet is extremely restricted. What would happen if the grocery store closed, and I couldn't get the few foods I lived on? I would … starve?

In many ways, the pandemic didn't touch my life the way it did my healthy friends' lives. Their responses troubled me more than the possibility of getting the virus. They said seeing fellow believers was essential to obeying God. They were certain they would rot at home.

That meant shut-ins were rotten, for sure. And yet, the general opinion is that shut-ins have a strong faith. Where do they get it?

"But your circumstances and ours can't be compared. You don't *feel* like going away," the healthy people want to argue.

That's correct. Not feeling well makes some aspects easier. But it also means we cannot be as active as the healthy. Besides giving up socialization, hobbies, and favorite foods, we no longer have strength and energy. We lose friends and are misunderstood.

When the pandemic forced the healthy people to stay home, they were not accused of being lazy or antisocial. Everyone was in it together. They weren't misjudged. They weren't misunderstood.

Or were they?

One evening in June, I read an essay about grief.[10] Life changes cause grief, the author wrote, and COVID-19 changed lives. Torn out of their familiar going-away world, many grieved. They ached for what used to be.

My eyes opened. I saw the truth: although some people *were* merely insubordinate to the government, others weren't. They felt misplaced and lost. Uncertainty gnawed at their heart.

I knew how it felt. As I remembered my experience, their words and emotions made sense. So why should I judge them? Why hurt them the way they hurt me?

It wasn't in my place to remind all the healthy people that, at last, they can find out what it is like to be homebound. I should reach out to them. Validate. Care. Encourage. Do what Jesus would do.

---

10   Ferree Hardy, "Some Good News for a Change," *Plain Values,* June 2020

Mask Confusion

Jane Weaver

MASKS COME IN all shapes and sizes, like the people who sew them. And the people who wear them—some most grudgingly, others with gusto.

My happy place is the Lancaster County store where I work. We sell lots of fabric, décor, and elastic. But then came COVID-19. It seemed as though the oceans had sneezed and infected millions around the world.

We stayed open as long as we dared and then closed for a week and a half, reopening again when masks were deemed essential. But it wasn't the same; our clientele had changed. People who had never sewn a seam arrived for supplies, armed with how-to instructions and a vague idea of what they needed. The masks they wore couldn't hide their desperation.

Every customer wanted yards and yards of elastic. So many yards of elastic! It wasn't unusual to measure twenty-five or fifty yards of elastic for one customer. It didn't take long to sell all the quarter-inch elastic we had. Several rolls of one-eighth-inch came to the rescue, but some customers were skeptical. Others tried cutting wider elastic in half lengthwise to get their desired width. Some bought bias tape to use as ties.

We sold all the plain black fabric we had on hand. One lady bought fifteen yards and wanted to order more. Someone bought all the solid brown fabric to make masks for the National Guard. We sold football- and baseball-team fabrics. Before we knew it, the Pennsylvania-sports-team fabrics were gone. Mary Jane ordered more, but she was told it would be June or July before it arrived. We sold fabric printed with doughnuts, dogs, cats, flip-flops, patriotic symbols—so much fabric and interfacing. Quarter-yard and half-yard cuts were the most popular.

One woman, tired of using up scraps, decided the residents at the nursing home would like nice masks. She chose light blue with muted swirls for the gentlemen, and a soft lavender print and one with bunches of pink flowers for the ladies. I could imagine folks chatting pleasantly through their masks, delighted to be out of the confines of their tiny rooms, glad to see their friends once again.

Another lady chose a variety of prints to make both masks and aprons for friends and family. "After all," she said, "everyone is spending more time in the kitchen."

"Call me Velveeta Cheese," a customer said, her words muffled by her mask. Her eyes sparkled, and her dark lashes, curled to perfection, contrasted with her light hair. "That's what my name sounds like." She searched the novelty section for just the right fabric to turn into masks, while I worked in the Christmas room, my mask under my chin. "Your smile is beautiful," she said with a wink. "We can't see that with these." She tugged her own mask down so I could see her smile.

At first when I asked how many masks they made, customers would reply with numbers somewhere between one hundred and four hundred, which seemed like a lot. This week a customer told me she had made five thousand. One lady planned to give any money she earned from selling masks to the food pantry.

There were always discussions as to whether the curved pattern gives more protection than a pleated-rectangle style. One customer bought Velcro to use on a bandana-type mask for construction workers.

Some people made cute masks for dolls, to match the ones little girls wore. I've sewn a dozen just for fun.

While a customer waited for me to cut the fabric she wanted, she asked if I personally knew anyone who had COVID-19. When I admitted I didn't, she told me about her ninety-three-year-old father, who had gotten sick. He lived in Vermont, and the hardest part was that his family could not go to be with him. Her eyes held weariness and grief. And I realized then how different the entire scenario would be if someone I loved were sick or dying from COVID-19.

One Saturday felt particularly hectic; the phone rang nonstop, and more people ventured out for supplies to sew masks. There was a continuous line at the cutting counter. I caught myself clenching my teeth behind my mask while I worked as fast as I could.

After the last customer left, we started cleaning up. I surveyed the shopping cart piled high with so many bolts of fabric that it slanted at a dangerous angle. There were bolts on the floor and bolts on the counter. So much disarray in one place!

"I hate elastic!" I proclaimed, startling my coworkers.

"But we do need it for some things," Lydia protested. "Maybe we should just go home and clean up this mess on Monday."

Shrugging, I kept stacking bolts to be put away. What if, as one man had said, wearing a mask was like putting up a chain-link fence to keep mice out? What if he was right?

Recently my friend told me about an encounter she had when she went to the grocery store. Kim, a friendly cashier with a personality that suits her flamingo mask, asked, "Is it your day off from the fabric store?"

Confused, it took my friend a moment to realize that Kim had mistaken her for me.

I laughed at the mix-up.

"It's time to get these masks off so people can know who's who," my friend added.

I wonder if our masks are hiding us more than helping us—disguising our personalities, along with our expressions. And it seems we've all lost our ability to hear.

But I find comfort in knowing that our Almighty Father sees past the masks and into our hearts; He never gets His children confused.

The Facing of This Hour

Erica Sauder

I SLOUCHED ON a patio chair at the Home on the afternoon of June 1 and closed my eyes, trying to shut out Kurt Morse, the in-house advisor and soon-to-be administrator. "It won't be that bad," he proclaimed. "You'll all look back on this with fond memories."

I work at the Gingerich Home for the Elderly in Farmington, New Mexico. Around the middle of March, we were required to ban all visitors from the Home in order to protect those in our care.

The Gingerich Home board asked those of us who worked at the Home not to do any shopping or visiting. The first couple of weeks dragged by, but I soon adjusted to a new normal, and time sped up again. Around the middle of May, we were given permission to go to town once a week. There were times I longed to be free to do what I wanted, free to go to town as much as I liked, free to visit friends, but for the most part, I didn't mind terribly.

Or rather, I didn't mind until June 1. That was the day of the first round of state-ordered COVID-19 testing. All the staff and all the ladies—our residents—had to be tested. Because the houseparents, Harley and Esther Mae Kauffman, were in contact with Home staff, they were also asked to get tested.

There was no way I could avoid the testing, short of losing my job.

A car rolled in the drive, followed by a van with a "State of New Mexico" seal on the driver's door. Three Department of Health personnel emerged, along with a stack of gear. Two of them traded homemade masks for medical ones and suited up in gowns, head caps, face shields, and two pairs of medical gloves, as though we were some sort of biohazard.

"Who's first?" asked the lady in charge of the test-kit file.

"I am," said Kurt. He told her his name, and she pulled his test kit from the file. He sat on the chair by the table and tilted his nose in the air. He grimaced as a technician plunged a long white swab deep into his nasal passage.

"Well!" Kurt said as he rose to his feet a few seconds later. "That was . . . wonderful." I didn't believe him; I doubt anyone else did either.

"Who's next?" asked the test-kit lady.

"Me," I said, determined to have the horrid thing over with before I watched too many others. I told the lady my name, and she pulled out my test kit and handed it to one of the technicians. Out came the long white swab, and up my nose it went. I gasped and squirmed, unable to sit still. It didn't take more than a few seconds, but oh, it was awful.

I tried to comfort the girls waiting to be swabbed, "It doesn't exactly hurt. It just burns, and feels *wrong*."

I hoped I wouldn't have to get tested again for several weeks. After the first round, we could go to percentage testing, with only three residents and two staff members getting tested every week.

I was thankful that I had received permission for a trip to Texas that weekend. I could get away from the stress for a few days and think about something else. I planned to enjoy my trip and not worry about the Home.

On the second day of my trip, I called the Home. "I'm at Walmart," I told Esther when she answered. "They have lots of disposable masks here. Fifty masks for thirty dollars—shall I get some for the Home?"

"Maybe you should. Harley tested positive, and now we all have to get tested every week. Since the ladies all have to wear masks to get tested, we might need more."

Every week? How could I possibly handle getting tested every week?

So much for not thinking about the Home while on my trip; now I could think of little else but the fate that awaited me when I returned. Skipping out on the second round of testing did little to console me; I would still have to get it done the next Monday, and the next, and the next . . . I was sure I couldn't handle it, but equally sure I could do nothing about it—other than have a breakdown, which I felt on the verge of.

I couldn't figure out why it was bothering me so much. The test took only a few seconds and didn't do any damage, but I couldn't talk myself out of my mental state. As much as I dreaded going back to New Mexico and to work, the day to fly back came. After several days of quarantining, I returned to work.

The following Monday I had the day off, but had to be at the Home by ten thirty to get tested. The week before, when I was in Texas, the test had been a throat swab. Some of the girls said it was much better than a nasal swab, but others said it had gagged them. I wasn't sure which test to dread, the nasal swab or the throat swab. I had tried hard to keep calm that weekend, but as I walked to the Home, my nerves hit my stomach. I relaxed a little after I joined the others awaiting the same torture.

The health department wanted us to stay farther away this time, so instead of gathering on the porch, we met in the dining room and had an impromptu staff meeting while we waited for the health-department personnel to suit up.

Which test would it be? If it was a nasal swab, the residents would need to wear masks, so Elizabeth—the supervisor—went out to ask. "It's a nasal swab," she announced.

"Let's watch Kurt get tested!"

I didn't join the girls crowding at the windows to see how Kurt reacted; I hated seeing it done about as much as getting it done.

"I don't think it's going in nearly as far!" one of the girls said.

"It looks like it's going in only about an inch instead of four inches."

"But they are doing both sides."

Really? I can handle that.

A few minutes later, I plopped in the testing chair and pulled my mask down off my nose. I eyed the swab coming my way, trying to see if it looked as long as the other one, but couldn't tell. But when the swab entered my nose, it felt much different. Instead of thrusting it halfway to my brain, the health-department lady stuck it just inside my nose and gave it a few twirls. After she repeated it on the other side, I was done. It had tickled but nothing more. *All that worrying and fretting for nothing!*

Because no one else tested positive, we were allowed to go to percentage testing the next week. I hoped to put off my turn for as long as possible. When Kurt asked for volunteers for the second week of percentage testing, I acted as if I hadn't heard what he said. Thankfully, two girls soon volunteered, and I didn't have to keep up the act for very long.

But within the next day or so, Kurt's wife, Naomi, came to me with a sheepish look. "Um, would you mind getting tested on Monday?"

"Do we need to do more than two?"

"No, Sheryl volunteered, but it's her day off. I don't want her to have to come in on her sleep-in morning."

I did mind, but this way I could get it over with for at least four weeks, maybe more. "I guess so," I told Naomi.

By this time, Basin Home Health was administering our tests, using throat swabs. I didn't think the throat swab could be too bad—surely my gag reflex wasn't that sensitive.

"Now this might gag you," warned the home-health lady as she advanced with a long swab.

Did you have to tell me that?

I opened my mouth, allowed her to depress my tongue with an icky wooden stick, and tried not to panic. As soon as the swab hit the back of my throat, I gagged and shoved her hand away from my mouth. She tried a second time, and I did the same thing. This time, though, she got a sufficient swab.

Four months later, we are still required to continue percentage testing. As much as I dislike being tested, it isn't nearly as bad as I had imagined it would be. God doesn't promise me grace for my imaginations, or even for tomorrow. But He does—and always will—provide what I need to face this hour.

Fear Hath Torment

Ruthanna Stoltzfus

ONLY A MONTH. Four short weeks until we would know. My stomach twisted with fear. Tears threatened to spill. Never in my wildest imaginations had I pictured missing our son's wedding! Our firstborn's at that. Of all the things I had worried about through his growing up years, this was not one of them. And certainly not because of a sickness. Only several months ago I had never heard the word *COVID*; now my whole world was turned upside down because of it.

My bare feet swished through the grass as I returned to the house, lugging my wash basket. Parrots screeched overhead as the sun set behind the elegant palm trees. If only my thoughts were as peaceful as the Bolivian countryside surrounding me. My mind traveled to our son and his bride-to-be thousands of miles away in Pennsylvania, where the wedding was to be held. If only I could fly like those parrots and be there tomorrow.

I flipped open the laptop. Maybe, just maybe, there would be an email from the American embassy, saying the country would open its borders before our date to fly. Copa Airlines had already canceled our tickets to fly up the month before the wedding. And now we were praying desperately that repatriation flights would be available before THE DAY arrived.

I could hardly bear to look at our wedding dresses hanging in the closet. What if we couldn't wear them to the big event? As the days crept by, I tried to act calm and happy for the children's sakes. I tried hard to remember that *all* things work together for good, but ugly fear kept creeping in. I pictured us listening to the wedding by phone, trying to envision the radiant bride and groom. My appetite was affected—who feels like eating with so much stress?

Finally, one day I spied it. An email from the American Embassy. My fingers fairly shook as I clicked on it. The delightful words leaped from the page. "Flights are available for American citizens." And before the wedding. Oh, what shouting and thanking God! We jumped in a vehicle and raced to our friend's house to buy tickets.

The day arrived to fly to the States. Only those with permits were allowed to drive to Santa Cruz, where the airport is. What would we do at the police checks? My husband printed out the airline tickets and stuck them with our passports in his briefcase. Sure enough, we were pulled over. The officer disappeared into the drab olive-green police shack, clutching our precious passports and tickets. Stressful minutes ticked by. "Please, Lord, don't turn us back now." Finally convinced we weren't lying, the officer let us continue.

Over an hour later, we arrived at Viru Viru airport. Everyone reluctantly pulled on a face mask. To enter the airport, we had to walk through a tent, dip our shoes in disinfectant, and get sprayed with strong-smelling liquid. A lady in what looked like a space suit took everyone's temperatures. The airport was a ghost town—only one international flight going out. All the restaurants were closed.

We walked to our gate and found out our flight would be taking off quite a while after our scheduled departure. Now what? Everyone was getting thirsty, but we had emptied our water bottles at security. I trudged through the airport searching. Surely one restaurant or store would be open. But no, there was no water to be bought. I returned from my futile trek and sank onto my hard seat again. Finally, one of the children discovered a little table with plastic cups filled with water. What a relief!

After long hours of waiting, we finally boarded. They announced we needed to wear our masks during the entire flight except when we were eating. My mask was securely on, covering my mouth, and I was sleeping deeply when a tap on my shoulder awakened me. "You must cover your nose also," reprimanded the tall flight attendant leaning over my seat. *Sigh...*

Finally, after two days of travel, we arrived in Washington, DC. We were delighted to finally be in the land of the wedding!

Now we could be at the special day, but what about the other three hundred fifty invited guests? Many weddings in recent months had been smaller, but now most couples were allowed full-sized weddings. Only a week before the big day, we heard that PA was again putting laws into place to limit the number of people at gatherings. My stomach knotted with familiar fear. Surely after so many prayers got us here, we wouldn't need to limit the wedding to family only. Thankfully, religious gatherings were exempt from the law, and we proceeded as planned.

The wedding was beautiful. All the more so because of the uncertainty we had experienced in getting there.

But would we be able to get back home? We, along with our nephew and niece, needed to be back for the first year of Bible school for our youth in Bolivia. Searching revealed we were able to fly home to South America on repatriation flights for Bolivian citizens. We happily purchased tickets. Only a few days before time to fly we received an email from the airlines with a list of requirements that were nearly impossible to fulfill.

We all needed negative COVID tests within seven days before we flew. Every place I called said, "It will be at least six to ten days till the results come back." I spent a good part of a day trying to find a place that would have a quicker turnaround. Finally, a hospital two hours away promised results in three to five days. Four days before our flight, we traveled the distance and all endured having a stick stuck up our noses till the tears ran. We filled out a stack of paperwork for each of us. Then we waited and prayed that the test results would be back within three days. To our amazement, the results were in the day before we flew. Every single one of them was negative.

Hurdle number two. We needed to send $250 per person to a Swiss bank account to reserve rooms for our week of quarantine at a luxury hotel in Santa Cruz. So, my husband made a trip to the bank and spent hours wiring money.

Our trip from Washington Dulles to Miami went well. In Miami, we had to fill out a mountain of paperwork for each passenger, including a hand-drawn map of where we lived. To spy on us in case we had the sickness? The lady at the desk checked carefully over our COVID tests. They all looked good except one. That test was taken in another state and didn't look as professional as the rest of ours. It was not acceptable. Now what? Leave our niece behind to get retested and fly later? After more prayers and some work on the laptop, the test was accepted. We all sighed with relief when we were finally on the plane headed to Bolivia.

The sun was just coming up over Santa Cruz as we trailed behind a porter pushing our mountain of luggage past a formidable row of policemen. No way to escape. We all were herded into a line of about eleven buses. Just up the road from the airport, the whole row pulled over into a grass strip along the road. For half an hour, we filled out more paperwork. The hotel where we would be quarantined for a week needed to know, along with many other questions, what kind of diet we preferred—bland, vegetarian, or normal. We sat and waited. And waited some more. Finally, the engines roared to life, and one by one the buses pulled onto the road and headed toward Los Tajibos Hotel. Except ours.

The driver cranked the key, but the bus sputtered and died. After several tries, the driver climbed out. Within minutes, a police bus came flying up beside us to see if we were trying to escape. We were exhausted from traveling for nearly twenty-four hours and longed for showers, a strong cup of coffee, and a soft bed. Everyone gathered up their bags and wearily climbed off the disabled bus and onto another one that had come to the rescue. Soon, we caught up with the rest of the buses, which had pulled over to wait for us, and the procession continued to the hotel.

Awful-smelling spray showered over us and our luggage as we entered the hotel. Every person was issued a separate room with a king-size bed. Our luggage filled one room. Several rooms we left empty, and the children paired up two to a room.

Three times a day, men looking like space aliens with suits, masks, plastic gloves, and protective glasses gingerly handed us our plates of food. Only one plate of food would be delivered to each room. As soon as we heard the wheels of the food cart coming, we ran like zoo animals at feeding time, each person standing at his "cage" door.

Once a day we were permitted outside on a section of lawn for exercise. Thankfully, we had aerobic rings and baseballs and gloves along. We made a lot of fun memories playing with other hotel guests.

I had prayed I could talk to someone about Jesus during our quarantine. And God sent a Lauren, a woman from Florida who was married to a Bolivian. By the time the week was over, we had become good friends. We discussed many topics in the exercise yard, including the way Mennonites dress, our school, and our choice to move to this foreign land.

The week dragged on with too much time for sleeping and eating. But we loved the extra hours for quality family time, devotions, reading, and singing. The evening before we were discharged into the real world, we all donned masks and took the elevator to the second floor. Chairs were spaced at six-foot intervals along the hall. We each found a chair and waited our turn to have our temperature taken and be declared COVID free.

The next morning, we were overjoyed to walk through the glass doors into sunlight and freedom. Home. Home, where our church brethren are not afraid. Where faith triumphs over fear. Where we keep having church and using the Christian greeting. A haven in a fear-crazed world.

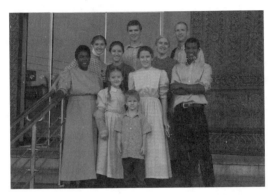

The Stoltzfus family: free to go home
after quarentine

Let Me Go Home

Faith Martin

"MOM TESTED POSITIVE for coronavirus," my husband, Delmar, told me over the phone.

My chest tightened with dread. "Are they sure?" I questioned. "How can they tell so soon? How can so quick a test be accurate?"

"I don't know, but they are making Dad leave the hospital."

"They are making him leave?" I was getting agitated. "What if she doesn't make it? Could he just take her with him?"

"She is miserable enough tonight Dad could hardly care for her at home. She needs to be in the hospital," my husband gently explained. "After ten days of quarantine, she can probably come home. Dad will also be quarantined."

"But she needs her husband!" I lamented. "Nearly three hours from home and so sick. How do they expect her to bear it alone?"

My husband's mother had battled multiple myeloma for nearly two years. She survived spinal surgery and, after recovery, did quite well on a low-dose chemo pill. But lately we had seen a gradual decline in her health. A month before, she had suffered an exhausting cough and had gone to the clinic to be tested for the coronavirus. The doctor ordered a flu test instead. That test was positive, so no further testing was done. In spite of her coughing, Mom busied herself organizing her closets and sorting items for a family garage sale. She was always tired, but her smile was bright.

Then Mom started having trouble with double vision. The eye doctor requested an MRI to see if a tumor could be causing it. The MRI appointment was scheduled in Columbia, two and a half hours from home. They left early in the morning, and since she was not allowed to eat, they fasted together. Before the MRI, she was tested for COVID.

The test was positive. The doctors decided she would not have an MRI that day. The trip, the hours of fasting, and the stress of a positive COVID test were too much for her weakened body.

The pain of the separation from her husband was much greater than her physical pain. Dad promised her she could call him any time of the day or night, and she did. The rest of us relied mostly on texting so we wouldn't disturb her rest.

Mom asked Dad for her Bible, so on the fourth day he went to the place where his dearest was confined. He left the precious package with the hospital worker who guarded the door, walked back to his vehicle, and drove home.

One night, Delmar couldn't sleep. Soon after midnight he got up and went outside for a prayer walk. As he walked out our long lane, he prayed for his mother. He pulled out his phone and sent her a text message. "Keep up your courage, Mom. I love you."

Her reply was instant. "I just dreamed I was in heaven. I want to go so bad."

Soon after that, she told Dad she wanted to be home, but not for long. She wanted to go to heaven.

Mom had been in the hospital for a week when our family pictures arrived in the mail. I wanted her to see them.

"Yes," Dad said, "she needs to have those pictures of her family hanging by her bed."

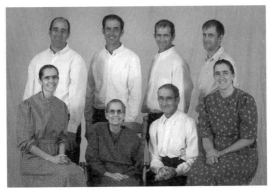

Edith Martin surrounded by her family
on Mother's Day 2020

I decided to take them to her on Saturday. "What if I would pretend I don't know better and ask to see her?" I asked Dad.

"You wouldn't get anywhere."

Dad picked a bouquet for me to take to her. He chose flowers and greenery from the hanging baskets, bushes, and flower beds around their porch. The bright blooms spoke of love and home.

Leaving early in the morning, I went alone. As I neared the hospital at eight o'clock, everything was eerily empty. I parked close to the entrance. Just as Dad had said, a table sat right inside the sliding door. Behind the table stood two workers wearing masks and gloves.

"May I help you?" A gentle voice banished my brief imaginations of a mad dash for the elevator.

Suddenly I was fighting tears. *This lady has an awful job.*

"Yes," I told her, "I have a few things for Edith Martin."

"I will see that she gets them right away," she told me kindly.

"Thank you," I whispered and turned to leave.

When I was back on the highway, I got a text message from Mom. "You are great!" she wrote.

"You are so worth it!" I sent back.

Three of Dad's six children spent Sunday evening with him. He built a fire in the backyard, and we all stayed outside. It was different to be at Mom and Dad's home without Mom. We talked about her hopes for coming home the next day.

On Monday morning, Dad prepared for Mom to come home. With great disappointment we heard that hospice would not be able to get all her equipment set up that day. She would have to wait till Tuesday.

Dad dreaded telling Mom the disappointing news, but to his surprise, she was prepared to accept it. "I decided it is very selfish of me to expect the hospice workers to put in overtime just so I can go home today," she said. "I can wait one more day." She was at peace—on Tuesday she was going home.

She came out of the ambulance waving jubilantly, her face beaming behind her oxygen mask. When they moved her into the living room, she motioned and pointed to her favorite chair. She was *not* going to the bed.

The medical personnel, in an unbelievable amount of protective gear, removed her mask and hooked her up to a nasal cannula. Now she could talk.

Because I was eager to go over, I thought I would mix up a batch of noodles and make the chicken soup she so loved for their supper. When I discovered I had used up the last of my chicken breasts, I decided to leave Mom and Dad alone together. "I will go tomorrow," I planned.

Around six thirty, Delmar messaged Dad. "How's it going?"

"Real good," came the answer.

My little girl had trouble going to sleep that night, so I slept in the girls' room. I was awakened by Delmar standing in the doorway.

"Mom passed away," he said softly.

Like a silent shot, I was beside him. "Are you serious?" I asked in an astonished whisper.

We moved into the bathroom to talk. Delmar didn't know much, just that Dad had gotten up to check on her, and she was gone.

I glanced at the clock. "It's not even midnight. He's there alone with her. Call him back and ask if you should come."

While Delmar made the call, I sent a message to our children. "Our sweet Grandma went to heaven."

DeLynn responded instantly, "No way. Grandma Martin?"

He then called and said he had passed their lane about five thirty. He had almost stopped in, but he decided to let her rest on her first evening home.

Dad said he didn't think Delmar needed to come, but he stayed on the phone for nearly an hour while waiting for the undertaker. While on the phone, Dad said that Mom had been so cheerful during the evening.

Mom ate her supper in bed. Then she said, "I can't go to bed if I don't get out of bed first."

Dad put her in her chair, but soon she just sat with her eyes closed, no longer talkative.

Poor girl, Dad thought. *She had a full day, so I won't weary her with talking. There's plenty of time for that tomorrow.*

"So," he said to Delmar, "I put her back to bed. She wasn't in bed long until she said she was having trouble getting her breath. Hospice had told me what to do if she gets that way, so I gave her morphine and a pill to relax her. I fanned her with a book for a while. Then I got a fan blowing over her, but she had no relief. I called hospice, and the nurse said to give another dose of medicine. So I did. That was about nine thirty. I told Mom, 'I'm so sorry, I just don't know what else to do.'

"She just motioned to me that it was all right. I prayed with her, and then said, 'I might just lie on the couch a little.' She motioned for me to go ahead. I lay down and prayed, *Lord, if it's not your will to relieve her, then just take her.* It still never entered my mind that she really was dying, or I would never have lain down," he said.

"Anyhow, I prayed hard, and in a short time, probably less than ten minutes, I thought, *Oh, Mom's not restless anymore. The medicine must be taking hold after all.* I thanked God for answering my prayer. In all reality, I think that is when He came for her. Oh," he grieved, "I can't believe I was in the room letting her die by herself!"

Dad told us later that he believes God didn't allow him to think he would lose Mom that first night so he wouldn't hinder Him when He came for her. This way Mom didn't have to struggle to leave him. "I feel it was of God," he said, "and I want to be satisfied with that. He makes no mistakes."

It was after four in the morning when Delmar and I went back to bed.

"You'll probably write a poem for her, won't you," Delmar said to me. It was statement, not a question.

"No," I told him. "I'm sure I won't."

After a few moments, I said, "If God gives me a poem, I will write it, but I don't have one."

Minutes later, while my husband slept soundly, my little light shone on my tablet, and my pen scratched snatches and lines.

Let Me Go Home
written from Mother's perspective

Oh, let me go home—my heart breaks for family,
To be with my husband again!
Our cabin, our haven, 'tis there I can rest
Surrounded by all that love brings.

These walls are my prison, I cannot go thither,
And neither can you come to me.
The law has forbidden that any should enter
To comfort and stand beside me.

They brought me my Bible, my own care-worn version.
I knew you had packed it with care,
And traveled the long road to stop at the entrance,
Then leave without seeing me here.

The pages bring comfort, God's truth now shines bright,
Assurance of His love and yours.
Dissolving the gloom and the chills of the morning.
This too shall pass—then I'll go home!

It's real! I am leaving my prison behind me,
I'm headed for home—my heart sings!
Our cabin, our haven, 'tis there I will rest
Surrounded by all that love brings.

I'm smiling, I'm waving, my husband to greet me,
He's here now to see me at last!
My chair—oh the comfort, my place at the table,
Our home is most surely the best.

But still I am weak, and my body is failing
I don't think I came home to stay.
My days here are numbered, my true Home is Heaven
And soon I am going away.

To Heaven, to Jesus, my parents, my sisters,
My heart longs for Heaven's release.
O let me go Home, to be healthy forever!
Surrounded by all that love brings.

Say *Grapefruit!*

Jacquie Hoover

WHEN I WAS young, my mom had a cure for all of life's little ailments. Spoken urgently, the implied meaning was clear: if not done immediately, it wouldn't work. When choking on a bite of food, we heard, "Put your arms up!" and if we skinned a knee, "Blow on it!" And my favorite: with the niggling of an impending sneeze, Mom would shout, "Say *grapefruit!*" Why the word *grapefruit* had power to stop a sneeze, I'm not sure, but once in a while it worked.

I haven't asked my mom what her cure for COVID-19 is, but I'm pretty sure she would say, "Wear a mask!" with the same urgency she used to say, "Put your arms up!"

So, I always carry a few masks with me just in case a sign on the grocery store door surprises me with "Masks required." I am not a mask person; they make me feel ill. But my daughter

Caroline is. At ten years old, she doesn't worry about having morning sickness and breathing her own stale air, or fogging up her glasses. She just wants to wear a mask because she thinks it's fun. Sort of grown-upish.

"They're all wearing masks, Mom," she warns as we swing into a parking spot at Aldi. Her voice sounds a tad hopeful, I think.

"Well…" I glance around, a tad hopeful myself, but for different reasons. "There's someone going in without a mask. Let's go."

Signs on the door urge, "STOP! Do not enter if you have a fever, headache, or cold." And, "Out of respect for our valued customers, please maintain social-distancing guidelines by keeping six feet between yourself and others at all times." Another one reads, "The CDC highly recommends wearing a mask to protect others from harmful transmission of disease."

Nowhere do I see the word *required*, so I enter.

The atmosphere in the store is tense. I feel the eyes of the CDC upon me and see the leery glances the masked shoppers cast my way. Not long ago, only robbers wore masks in stores. Now I'm the felon, the unmasked one about to rob people of their health. Uneasily, I check items off my list. Graham crackers. Tortilla chips. Bread.

Before COVID, I never thought much about rummaging through the produce, but now I wonder if the person standing six feet behind me is worrying about the germs I leave on every cucumber I touch. I make a hasty selection and move on to the tomatoes. *Maybe I should have worn a mask; others might consider me disrespectful.* I nestle a tomato in my cart next to the lettuce, and ponder this. I certainly don't want to be disrespectful.

I reach for a bag of onions, but a tickle in my nostrils stops me. The feather of a sneeze twists in my nose. I wiggle it rabbit-style, and the sting subsides, then surges. If I rub my nose, do I continue using my contaminated hand? The delinquent sneeze torments me while my mind grasps at options. If inevitable, do I stuff my nose into my elbow and sneeze *away* from the produce? What about the people standing six feet on either side of me? Should I sneeze *facing* the produce? I imagine masked gasps, and then the manager escorting me out of the store while an employee in full PPE scoops the contaminated produce into a trash bin.

If only I could sneeze like my sister! We have the same size nose, but her single-syllable *choo* is kept mostly confined, executed so daintily that most people aren't even aware of what just happened. I, on the other hand, sneeze with gusto, a gale-force *kerchoo!* meant to get the job done.

So I trundle down the produce aisle, fighting the flickering sparks burning in my nose. I am studying the cabbages when the sparks burst into flame, and I make a decision: I will seal my lips together—sort of hold it back—and hope for the best.

What comes out sounds like a trumpet blown between two pieces of plastic.

Caroline's head snaps up, questions all over her face. *What was that noise?*

"I had to sneeze," I whisper. The sound replays in our minds, an off-kilter bellow in an off-kilter world, and we are struck silly. Is laughing allowed? By all appearances, it is not, so we duck down the potato-chip aisle to gasp out our giggles.

"Mom," Caroline chides, "you should have worn a mask."

No. I should have said *grapefruit.*

Of COVID and Cookies

Joel Showalter

AFTER MORE THAN five months of lockdown, the streets of Tegucigalpa remain relatively empty. It definitely curtails normal business when each person is permitted to circulate only one day out of every two weeks.

A bumpy, washed-out section of highway on the outskirts of the city slowed the vehicles so much that the line of traffic was backed up for a couple of miles. It was four in the afternoon, and I was eager to get home. But all I could do was follow the endless pattern: surge ahead, slow down, stop. It was almost like old times to be stuck in a traffic jam.

After a while, I noticed a couple of people in the road ahead. Nothing unusual in Honduras, especially during the COVID crisis. Many hungry citizens have taken to begging from the passing travelers. Inching closer, I could see that these two were young girls, one on either side of the line of traffic.

The one on the right, who appeared to be about fourteen, held a dilapidated shovel. Their strategy consisted of throwing an occasional shovelful of dirt into a pothole in the middle of the road while importuning the passengers of the slow-moving vehicles. The girl standing on the driver's side barely reached the bottom of my window. She might have completed eight or nine summers. A dirty yellow sweatshirt, pink pants, and raggedy cloth mask pulled under her tiny chin made up her costume. She scampered around in the center of the highway between the opposing lines of cars and trucks.

As I advanced cautiously between the girls, I lowered my window and looked directly into the eyes of the little one. I saw no fear, no guilt, no shame. Only expectant curiosity. Would this blue-eyed foreigner give her anything? She carefully pulled her cute little mask up over her mouth and nose. She could follow the rules even while she begged.

My recent custom has been to stock up on strawberry-jam cookies at the grocery store to bestow a treat on the needy instead of giving them money. Reaching into my bag, I pulled out a pack of cookies and handed them to the little girl. Eagerly she stretched up to grab the package, not sure what she was getting, just determined to capture all she could.

She turned the gift over. Then it registered. *Cookies!* Such a look of sheer delight illuminated that chubby, grubby, rosy face. She clutched the precious package to her chest in an ecstasy of satisfaction. Watching in my mirror, I saw her dancing in the center of the road, delighted over her treat.

COVID may have taken money from her family and forced her into the streets, but it couldn't take the simple joy of cookies. Small pleasures are great treasures to the impoverished.

Return to Normal?

Diane Kaufman

WHAT'S THE RUSH?
I'm still considering which parts of "normal,"
    if any,
        are worth rushing back to.
Do I wish to return to my Old Normal
    of the two weeks before COVID-19
    scared us all into quarantine?
  Back then,
    we held a memorial service for Sasha,
        with five hundred friends
      who gathered to mourn our loss with us
      in one large room.
  That weekend,
    we hosted a family of eight at our house,

in addition to the six of our family,
eating our meals together
around one big table.
The following week, on Thursday morning,
I got up early to bake twelve cups of rice
to serve with the Chipotle chicken
we had made for hot lunch at school,
preparing to serve
fifty students, teachers, and patrons
in one small room.
The next week, on Tuesday evening,
we hosted the local ministers' meeting
at our house,
with the ladies visiting upstairs
and the men meeting downstairs
in my husband's small office.
The next day, which was Wednesday,
I took my daughters and daughter-in-law
for a normal day of shopping.
But at Sam's Club, I was amazed
to find the pallets empty of rice and beans.
My daughter-in-law looked for toilet paper
and found *none* on the usual stack.
We were blissfully ignorant
of the approaching pandemic.
But that night, we learned
that the first four cases of The Virus
had been confirmed in our county.
Then we understood.
Saturday noon I took my husband

to the airport in Durango, Colorado,
for his flight to Alberta, Canada,
    where he was going to preach
    a series of revival meetings
        each evening
        for a whole week.
            Or so we thought.
            Or maybe it was just *hoped*.
On Sunday, I went to church
    without my husband.
On Monday, I took supper to a busy mother.
By Wednesday morning,
    I was on the way to the airport again,
        going to pick up my husband,
        who had preached
            just one revival message.
At midnight,
    the Canadian border closed
    to US citizens.
By the next week,
    we had started a New Normal.
The Lamp and Light Publishers'
    semi-annual board meeting
    was canceled,
        meaning no overnight guests
        or the traditional Thursday evening supper
        at our house.
The deacon ordination planned for that weekend
    was postponed till a later date.
        Again, we had no guests.

All the planned church services
were canceled.
Going to the Nationwide Ministers' Meetings
in Plad, Missouri, the following Monday morning
was no longer even a possibility;
those meetings were canceled, too.
School was canceled.
Suddenly, we were on lockdown,
warned to stay home
except for essential business.
I loved it—
more than most people seemed to.
Now I could stay home without feeling guilty.
For one whole week,
I did not go anywhere.
And every evening we were all at home.
Every one of us.
For one whole week.
There were no youth activities,
no meetings,
no guests,
nor any church services.
Each evening, we gathered in the living room
for family time.
Ah, how I reveled in this New Normal,
unprecedented for our family.
Finally, we could dig out the stories
we had been saving to read aloud.
We had time for unhurried family worship
and prayer times.

We could enjoy blackberry smoothies
  for bedtime snacks together.
I loved the New Normal of our daytime hours, too.
  Suddenly we had time for projects
    that had lain dormant for months.
  The Southwest quilt I had pieced
    for an older son
    was one of those projects.
  I had hoped to teach my younger children
    the art of quilting
    when I put the quilt in the frame
      ten months before.
Now we could uncover the quilt top,
    taking off the sheet
    that had been protecting the quilt
      from dust.
And leave the sheet off for days at a time.
Because now I could require my daughters
    to quilt for at least thirty minutes
      every day (except Sundays, of course)
      week after week.
My children learned to quilt,
    even my son (the youngest one).
      What's more, they learned to enjoy it.
One project completed.
Then my great-uncle died in Virginia.
  He was the last of my grandfather's generation—
    a smiling, jolly fellow
    whom many people lovingly called
      "Uncle Nelson,"

although they were not related to him
by blood ties.
In the twenty years we have lived
in this desert place,
we have traveled east
for only one family funeral—
to that of my Grandmother Vera.
Aunts and uncles have passed away since,
but it never suited for us
to make that long trip east
to grieve with the extended family
in their loss.
However, I had hoped
that when Uncle Nelson passed away,
we could attend his funeral
and grieve with the family in person.
But Uncle Nelson died in May,
right during the pandemic.
Because of COVID restrictions,
there could only be a graveside service
for immediate family.
I could not go to his funeral after all.
For the first time,
I understood on a heart level
why some folks hate quarantines
and social distancing
and state lockdowns.
Well, in truth, that was not quite the first time
this pandemic touched a heart chord of mine.
I had a little grandbaby I could not see,

much less hold,
even though she lived just a few miles away—
for one week,
then two weeks.
There was also a big sister at the same house.
After one week,
her grandpa and I drove up to their house
and waved to her
through the living room window.
After two weeks,
I could not stand it any longer.
This time, when I went to her house,
she sat on the front porch steps
and watched...
while Grandmother blew bubbles in the wind
from six feet away.
Now we act "normal" again,
when I go to their house
or when they come to mine.
That is a part of the Old Normal that I like.
I'm still considering if there are any other parts
of the Old Normal I wish to return to.
Yes, for my family's sakes, I believe there are.
My husband
would like a normal work atmosphere,
where all the employees
can work there at once
and enjoy normal break times
(everyone in the same room
at the same time),

and with all foreign mail
being delivered and received.
My older son
wishes for a normal courtship,
with more than once-a-week
phone calls and emails,
a courtship without an international border
separating him and his girlfriend,
keeping them from visiting together
face to face.
My schoolteacher daughter
longs for a normal school year,
one where she can teach her students
in a classroom,
rather than from a phone
at a table in her bedroom,
a whole school term of being able
to release in full
her passion for teaching
and her love
for the little people in her life.
My teenage daughter
longs for normal church life,
not just sitting at home for services,
listening to the sermon by phone,
or sitting in our vehicle
in the lower church parking lot
for a drive-up service
where the preacher stands behind a pulpit,
set on the hillside for his platform

with the trees on the lawn for his shade,
or even meeting in the church house
with only twenty-five percent
of the people present,
sitting by families
on every other bench,
but *real* church,
with everyone there,
including all her friends,
to worship God together.
My youngest son
wishes for a normal day
of selling produce at the farmers market.
You know, like it used to be
in previous summer seasons—
without ropes for social distancing,
or gloves for handling the produce
and even the money,
or hand sanitizer,
or face masks.
(Perhaps I should mention
this son is fifteen years old.)
Today at church,
with only twenty-five percent
of the congregation present,
the preacher referred to a plaque he saw recently
but did not purchase
because it portrayed such a feeling of doom.
The plaque listed a bunch of things
gone haywire in our world

because of this virus.
The concluding lines read,
"Due to a downturn in our economy,
and in order to conserve energy,
the light at the end of the tunnel
has been turned off."
Is there truly no hope of returning to normal?
For the Christian, some things stay the same,
or "normal,"
even in a pandemic,
since Jesus is still the same today
as He was yesterday.
Due to our trust in Him,
we can see light at the end of this tunnel!
Little by little,
life for me is starting to get some normalcy to it.
In many ways, I am glad.
But perhaps this whole time of upheaval in our world
and in our schedules
and in our plans,
yea, even in our daily lives,
has given us opportunity to consider
which parts of our old "normal"
are truly worth returning to.

—Written August 30, 2020

Pandemic of Opinions

Dorothy Swartzentruber

"I'VE SAID IT once and will say it again: unplug the phone, shut off your computer, stay at home, don't listen to what the neighbor reports from TV, and coronavirus is dead. I'd like to know why so many Mennonites are trying so desperately to stay out of heaven. They're gossiping full-time and believing the media instead of the Bible."

I read the email thoughtfully. Yes, I agreed that media hype instills fear rather than empowering people with faith. Yes, I agreed that many stories we were hearing could be rumors. Some had been proven false already. Yes, we Mennonites are quick to share what we hear with each other. But why did I feel uncomfortable about the spirit driving the words?

"It's absolutely crazy. The whole world has lost their heads over this. Christians shouldn't be acting so scared. We're following the world in fear! We should just go on living like normal, instead of losing our heads like everybody else."

I blinked. I had thought I was keeping a level head; I was not buying more groceries or toilet paper than usual. I reread the email. Once again, though I agreed with some of it, something felt muddy. After some thought I asked, "So you're saying that obeying these new laws is an act of fear?"

Yes, I had understood right.

I waited some time before attempting a reply. "Didn't God call us to respect and obey the law unless it contradicts Scripture? I agree, Christians should not fear the virus or death. But if this virus is even half as bad as some of the things I have heard, if I would help to spread it to someone who would then die from it, would that be right? The fact is that we do not know yet how serious this virus is. Until we know, I think God wants us to obey the government."

The next email from this person included a long list of Bible verses intended to support a courageous stand against the world during this pandemic.

She handed me the package she had brought. "It seems so long since I have seen you! Do you feel as starved for fellowship as I do? This just can't be right, this not having church," she said. "The Baptist church down the road has kept on having normal services the entire time. You know the Bible says we shouldn't forsake the assembling of ourselves. This sitting at home listening to services over the phone is not right."

Once again I was at a loss for words. After a few seconds of thought I ventured, "I know we can't understand why everyone is making the choices they are, but God calls us to respect authority. We don't need to understand to respect."

"Oh yes, we do respect our leaders," she assured me. "But it's not right for us to stop having church. We're starving spiritually because we're giving Satan the upper hand through obeying orders given in fear."

My neighbor lady raised her eyebrows and fired a question that sounded more like a statement. "You *are* going to wear a mask, aren't you? I sure don't want you going to the city and dragging germs back here to us."

I blinked. Wearing a mask hadn't even crossed my mind. They weren't mandatory in our state at the time. Now that I had heard from some COVID-19 survivors who didn't consider the symptoms extremely serious, I felt less concerned about taking precautions than I had.

"You will, won't you?"

I shrugged. "I might."

Her eyes nearly popped out of her head. "Don't be irresponsible, honey. You've got to do your part; we all do. It's part of following the Golden Rule."

Opinions, opinions. They became a pandemic right along with the virus. They flew farther and multiplied faster than any germ could, thanks to virtual communication.

Some people claimed the virus was a hoax. Some believed it came from eating bats. Some said it was spread by airplanes flying over. Others were convinced it had been created in an American lab and then sent out by China. Still others declared it was an end-times plague—the judgment of God on evil nations.

On the heels of those assessments came opinions on authority, respect, fear, and wisdom. Folks who questioned the wintegrity of the authorities' decisions felt comfortable with ignoring their laws. Some touted conspiracy theories. Some seemed to be motivated by a desire for their views to be proven right and for the views of others to be proven wrong. Other people appeared calm, not fearful, but serious about doing their part. During the time of size-limited public gatherings, some disregarded the law while other households restricted themselves to seeing no one.

The odd thing was that nearly everybody found Scriptures to prove their point. Opposing views were often supported by similar verses.

Where did we stand in all of this? Uncomfortably in the middle, treading softly in an apologetic effort to offend neither group. We could understand most folks' reasoning, but nobody thought exactly alike. In light of our own views, we made the choices that seemed wisest and quietly went about our lives, glad to allow everyone else the same liberty.

But what should we do when people tried to force their thinking onto us? How should we relate to people who considered themselves right while ridiculing the government and anyone who tried to obey the law? This challenge strung my nerves tight.

After listening to many opinions, trying to explain our view to some who thought differently, and being severely reprimanded for thinking the way we did, we discussed this problem with another couple. We concluded it's best to say as little as possible when COVID-19 is discussed. We wouldn't allow adamant opinions to sway us, but neither would we try to convince others to think the way we did. Even if some seemed to have a critical or scoffing spirit, we didn't need to point out their error. After all, "A man convinced against his will is of the same opinion still."

Whether that was always the wisest choice, I cannot tell. But our conclusions brought me a measure of peace when more loud opinions met my ears and eyes. Time would tell who was right; now was not the time to try to prove that, without hindsight to guide us. God has the patience of eternity. He doesn't need us to jump up and down, getting hyper when others disagree with our interpretation of His Word.

The first couple of lines from a Luci Shaw poem often came to mind:

I will not prevaricate—
Truth will out.

When the difference between opinion and truth is obscure, we can be assured of this: No virus—nor opinions about a virus—will ever change truth. In His time, God will show the truth, and no man will contradict it.

A List of Blessings in the Midst of a Pandemic

Phyllis Eby

I AM GRATEFUL to be the child of a King Who is bigger than anything in this world, Who is not taken by surprise by any pandemic or any government's response thereto, and Who has a plan for His children. I praise Him for the peace of His presence.

I am thankful to be part of a kingdom that is not threatened by COVID-19 or by changes and failures of earthly governments. When men's hearts are failing because of fear, I can stay my heart on Jehovah and know He will enable His army to go forward, no matter what the enemy may throw our way.

I am glad that when the Apostle Peter said, "Honor the king," he didn't ask us to first decide whether the king is corrupt, or whether he is making wise choices. I am glad I am not burdened with the huge decisions facing governments today. I am also thankful I don't need to lose sleep trying to decide what the results of those decisions will be.

Regardless what the future of this country may be, I am glad for the history of God's people who have been faithful under many kinds of unfriendly governments. I rejoice that the same God stands ready to give us grace should we need to face persecution.

I am awed that when we choose to honor the government as far as possible, regardless of corruption and poor decisions, that honor strengthens the foundation of our children's respect for our authority.

I am thankful that since our treasure is in heaven, a collapse of this country's economy, while it may make life here more difficult, cannot change our real net worth.

I am glad Christ invites us to seek the Truth which will make us free, not the truth about what is really going on in the world.

I am glad for physical health for myself and my loved ones and pray that it would continue. But I am even more thankful to know the Great Physician, Who has delivered me from the pandemic of sin. If COVID strikes us, I can trust Him to heal us or to take us to heaven.

I am grateful, I say softly, that our parents and grandparents are in good health so far, and we have not needed to make difficult decisions about traveling during this time.

I am so thankful that our congregation has found a way to gather in small groups for worship. But I am also thankful that even when we worshipped alone as a family or with a few other believers, the Spirit of God was with us. He accepted our worship, and our souls were fed, even in these less-than-ideal circumstances.

I am thankful we can find ways to fellowship even when we are absent one from another. I am glad for the ways our brothers and sisters have supported us with phone calls, emails, prayers, soup, granola, and patches sewn on little boys' pants.

I am glad we can trust that our brothers and sisters are seeking God's will and are led by His Spirit, even when their decisions differ from the ones we make.

Thinking of the millions required to stay at home in crowded cities, I am glad for plenty of outdoor space where our children can stretch their legs. I rejoice in fresh air, sunshine, and the privilege of growing things in the garden; there we gain exercise and emotional health.

When I hear of a sister in Peru leaving her home for the first time in a month, of young men in Paraguay getting stopped fifteen times on an essential five-hour trip, or of stringent restrictions in other countries, I am grateful for the mobility we have.

When I learn of the plight of people in many countries who live on day-to-day incomes, and who are now facing starvation because of being required to stay at home, I am almost embarrassed by our wealth. I give humble thanks for all the food on our shelves, for money to buy more when it is needed, and for available supplies, even though they may sometimes be hard to find.

I am especially indebted to the friends through whose prayers God is granting grace to deal with all the extra challenges of this time.

For all these blessings, Lord, and many more that slip my mind, I give You grateful praise. Thank You for bringing us closer to You through the unexpected happenings of this year.

Acknowledgments

ONE OF THE most enjoyable aspects of compiling this book was collaborating with others. I've had so much help from so many people, and I am so grateful.

Stephanie J. Leinbach, Sheila Petre, Gina Martin, Darletta Martin, and Stephanie A. Leinbach: Thank you for giving me the encouragement to pursue this project. Thank you also for answering my questions and giving me advice.

Darletta Martin: Thank you so much for helping with the editing. I enjoy working with you.

The writers: Without you, this book wouldn't exist. Thank you for trusting me with your words.

Christine Laws, Shawn Schmidt, and Stephanie Shirk: Thank you for all the hours you spent copy-editing, and for meeting my deadline.

Austin Witmer: Thank you for teaching me InDesign, and for patiently answering all my questions. Thank you also for doing the pre-press review.

Samuel Coon: Thank you for the review work you did. And for the advice.

Jonas and Judi Zimmerman and Cassie Yoder: Thank you for helping me finalize the story order.

Dad and Mom: Thank you for your support.

The many who aren't listed here but answered questions and gave advice, or just listened to me talk about this project: Thank you all so much.

Writers' Profiles

Marlene Brubacher

Marlene Brubacher lives among the mines and pines of northwestern Ontario where winters dip to -45 C, and summers echo with loons' yodels on sparkling lakes. She is a cleaner and baker who thrives on coffee, poetry, and global friendships. She helps edit a free monthly e-zine for Anabaptist missionary women; contact her at truthandwrite88@gmail.com for more info.

Megan Byler

Megan Byler is a twenty-year-old girl happily teaching at her home church in Hudson, New York, and is also the big sister to six brothers and sisters.

Deborah Coblentz

Deborah Coblentz was born in Wisconsin, spent her school years in Kentucky, and moved to Iowa as a teenager. But she celebrated her sixth birthday during her family's stint on a Costa Rican chicken farm, to which she credits her fascination for the Spanish language and Latin culture (though she developed no lasting affinity with the hens). Now a resident of Paraguay, she relishes the challenges involved in teaching, language study, and cross-cultural relationships, though frustration occasionally fringes the fascination.

Lavina Coblentz

When Joseph and Lavina married in February, 2014, in southern Iowa, and moved across the state line into northern Missouri, they never dreamed God would lead them to Paraguay, South America. God richly blessed their home with four children. They enjoy their small dairy, the Latin culture, and visitors.

Phyllis Eby

Phyllis Eby lives with her favorite preacher and their five children in southern Arizona. The three years since they moved here have changed their piece of desert into a home. They have also deepened her faith in the unfailing grace of God for every day. Becoming a better wife and mother is a full-time job, but she treasures moments with friends both old and new--whether they be people, books, or songs—as well as chances to introduce them to each other.

Laura Hawbaker

Laura Hawbaker is the wife of one, mom of eight, and grandma of an ever-expanding tribe. Laura and her husband of over forty years live near Dallas Center, Iowa. Laura loves words, whether it's reading them or writing them. She has randomly published in the past and is eager to dust off the keyboard and get back into writing again.

Jacquie Hoover

While Jacquie Hoover looks forward to the day when she can see people smiling in the grocery store again, her six young children remind her of the need for a merry heart at all times. She lives with her little posse and husband, Michael, in an old brick farmhouse in northern Indiana. You can reach her at behooved09@yahoo.com or 16407 County Rd. 52, Syracuse, IN 46567. A letter in either mailbox will be sure to make her smile.

Kristen J. Horst

Kristen fights an irresistible attraction to the library five minutes away, often succumbing to including it on her road trips. Tweaking recipes to try new flavors or to use what's on hand causes her husband to question whether she ever follows an original recipe. She married Kraig two years ago at age twenty-four and has encountered the love and pain of motherhood with the advent of Mitchell. She resides at 14286 Wingerton Rd, Waynesboro, PA 17268, and answers calls to 240-527-5099. She savors the flavor of grilled chicken, thrills to deep discussions, and enjoys making new friends and hosting company. To most folks she's just Kristen, but she adds J. Horst to clarify her identity.

Shannon Hostetler

Shannon Hostetler is a wife, mom, and a catch-all for all the things everyone else needs to have done. Her writings usually happen with a sudden burst of inspiration and a few scribbled notes, followed by a late-night writing session after her children are all in bed. Someday she dreams of having more time to write, but until then her rambles can be found at shannonhostetler.wordpress.com

Diane Kaufman

Diane Kaufman's life is full and fulfilled as a wife of one, mother of seven, and grandmother of eight favorite little people. She enjoys quilting, genealogy, and a good book. After COVID restrictions are past, you are welcome to spend a night in her guest bedroom, but you will need to make your own coffee in the morning!

Lucinda Kinsinger

Lucinda J Kinsinger lives in Oakland, Maryland, with Ivan, the love of her life. She is the author of *Anything But Simple: My Life as a Mennonite* (Herald Press, 2017) and *The Arrowhead* (Christian Light Publications, 2017), with several more books forthcoming. She writes a column for *Anabaptist World* and blogs at lucindajkinsinger.com.

Hertzen Kruse

Hertzen Kruse, a lifelong lover of all things literary, was born in 1990. She presently hails from northern Wisconsin, where the winters sometimes grow wearisome and spring is always a reason to celebrate. She is a complicated mixture of introvert and extrovert, thriving on both social gatherings and solitude. She loves bare feet, books, time with nieces and nephews, shades of turquoise, and chocolate. Trips to Paraguay, Canada, and California awakened her adventurous streak, and she dreams of opportunities to explore more of the world. Years of singlehood and school teaching have been a mixture of lessons on independence and dependence on the One she strives to glorify. She's always interested in expanding her circle of friends (especially writers), so feel free to contact her at N3565 Polar Rd. Bryant, WI 54418 or hk90@norcell.us.

Stacey LaSee

Stacey LaSee is a young lady from Wisconsin, who, in addition to doing in-home care and teaching violin and piano lessons, is passionate about youth ministry, music, and writing. Her desire is to live a life of service to God and others, bringing glory to her Creator.

Stephanie A. Leinbach

Stephanie had taught school for almost seven years when Naaman Leinbach ended her career by asking for her friendship. They were married the first day of 2005 and celebrated fifteen years together before they ever heard of COVID-19. The pandemic changed little for them since Stephanie homeschools their eight daughters (ages 4-14) and her husband works at an essential business, the mechanic shop across the road. They enjoy hosting friends and family from all over the United States who travel through their home territory, the Crossroads of America, but that came to an abrupt halt for a few months during the shutdown. Stephanie loves to hear from her readers. If you wish to contact her, you may email her at inleinbachs@gmail.com.

Stephanie J. Leinbach

Stephanie and Linford live with their four children—Jenica, Tarica, Micah, and Gairett—in a 1930s mountain home built by a Pennsylvania Railroad carpenter. In addition to history, architecture, and trains, she enjoys words, solitude, chocolate, and research. Connect with her at stephaniejleinbach@gmail.com.

Diane Martin

Diane Martin was born in 1978. She lives with her husband Allan and six children near Mount Forest, Ontario. They are part of the Markham-Waterloo Mennonite Conference.

Darletta Martin

Darletta Martin lives with her husband, Delmer, and two sons on a farm near Smithsburg, Maryland. Their other three children and six grandchildren live nearby. Her days are filled with homemaking, relating to family and friends, writing, editing, and baking. She has been richly blessed by God's grace, especially during the COVID season.

Faith Martin

Faith Martin lives with her loving husband in a big yellow farmhouse in the northeast corner of Missouri. The house built in 1917 was almost completely renovated before the Martins bought it in 2015. Faith's first love is mothering. She and her husband became foster parents at the age of twenty-one. The first child in their home was adopted three years later. More than forty children have known her love and called her Mom. She considers it the world's highest honor to have borne into the world two biological sons. Two more sons and a daughter were adopted internationally. Faith considers adoption a double miracle and will never take their U.S. citizenship for granted. The Martins also have two daughters-in-heart who lived with them most of their lives but to which they have no legal parenting rights. Faith counts them along with her children bringing the number to eight. Three of the eight are still at home. Her latest thrill is that of being "Grammy." Her grandson Kai is a year old and a joy to all the family. Over the years whenever she had spare time, Faith would be sewing. She also enjoys writing. In the throes of foster parenting many were the times she'd turn to her keyboard for release. She loves to share real life stories. Her heart's desire is that by her written words others may be drawn in to experience God's love. Her goal is to write so they may see His faithfulness and believe His truth.

Kervin Martin

Kervin Martin grew up in Myerstown, Pennsylvania, the youngest in a family of eight. He is currently in his third year of teaching school in Tabio, Colombia, South America. He has a passion for learning, with particular interests in Biblical studies, apologetics, issues facing the Church, all things science, wildlife, music, writing, languages, and of course, teaching. His life's goal is to inspire others to be dedicated to the work God calls them to.

Luke Martin

Luke had lived in three countries by the time he got married in 2015. He currently lives in Peru with his radiant wife, Grace, and three children, Luana Grace, Lia Shalom, and Kaspar Luke. Luke is a school teacher, which he says is an ideal job because it combines his passions for learning about the world and influencing lives for God's kingdom. It also gives him an excuse to travel, which he does whenever he can. In the meantime, he reads travel guides as a hobby and plans more excursions than he and his family will ever be able to take.

Sarah Martin

Sarah Martin lives in the rocky, tree-studded hills of Bancroft, Ontario with her stable, dependable husband, Edward, and their seven lively children. Next to raising her family and writing, Sarah enjoys photography. Sarah loves God, good music and literature, old churches, the smell of old books, and light in all its forms.

Rhoda Mazelin

Rhoda Mazelin lives in Missouri, where rolling landscape, sunrises, rainbows, family, and God's goodness bring joy to her life. Though struggling with ill health for a decade, she considers herself blessed.

Kurt Morse

Kurt P. Morse was born in western New York and spent his first fifty years there. After losing his first wife, Sheila, he moved to NC, where he lived for ten years. Currently, he lives in NM, where he married his second wife, Naomi. He is the father of four and grandfather of sixteen. Among other activities, Kurt has been a corrections officer, dairy farmer, sawmill operator, boys' home counselor, print shop worker and currently, Care Home administrator (something he never imagined doing). He is happiest when he is studying church history and encouraging others to follow God.

Naomi Morse

Naomi (Martin) Morse was born in PA, where she spent her first twenty-seven years, before moving to Farmington, NM. Naomi has had work experience in varying fields, including bulk foods and bakeries, teaching school, and working with the elderly. Her favorite job began in Jan. 2018, when she became the wife of Kurt Morse. Since their marriage they have spent a term of service at a boys' home in PA and are currently administrators at the Gingerich Home for the Elderly, where she worked for almost twelve years before her marriage. She enjoys cooking, knitting, talking, and occasionally writing.

Hannah Myers

Hannah (Burkholder) Myers was born near Chambersburg, Pennsylvania. On the evening of her first birthday, she took her first tottery steps alone when her family visited another church family one spring evening in May of 1973. Surely—I hope!—she played with their blond-haired, brown-eyed little cutie, only six months her senior. Two years later, the little boy moved with his family to Paraguay, South America. But ten years after that, Hannah remembers noticing him when as a teenager, he visited the community of his birth during a year-long sojourn in the U.S. Another eight years and the young man—now of age—returned to the country of his kindred, seeking work. (Did he have in mind to look for a wife?) God directed him to his "missing rib" and on October 28, 1995, she filled the gap next to his heart, where she's happily stayed ever since. Josiah and Hannah enjoyed their first three years of married life in

Somerset County, Pennsylvania, where a baby boy, Jordan Hays, joined their union. In September of 1998, they flew to Paraguay—Hannah had promised Josiah on their first date to accompany him there should the Lord direct that way—to establish a home in Colonia Florida. During the next thirteen years, God blessed them with seven more children— Jaleesa Wren, Heather Fawn, Sharla Gwen, Jenna Floe, Shannon Lane, Stanley Roye, and Harmony Brook. Family comes first, but Hannah's hobbies include writing, sewing, and painting. Her favorite verse always has been, is, and—I think!—always will be: "Jesus Christ the same yesterday, and to day, and for ever." (Hebrews 13: 8).

Sara Nolt

Sara Nolt is the wife of John and the mother of three extraordinary children. They live in a little yellow house in Stevens, PA, one situated close enough to the road that passersby can wave to them at the kitchen table. Homeschooling, freelance writing, and a never-ending laundry pile fill Sara's days while God and His eternal purposes fill her heart. You can contact Sara at johnandsaranolt@gmail.com.

Sheila Petre

Sheila shares love, laughter, and the hope of the resurrection with her husband, Michael, in a small house humming with children (nine) and words (more than they can count). They publish *The King's Daughter*, a quarterly periodical for young women. Sheila compiled *Vignettes*, a directory of Anabaptist women writers, and is the author of *Thirty Little Fingers*, a collection of her motherhood-related essays, poems, and stories. Reach her at P.O. Box 127, Mercersburg, PA 17236.

Mabel Reiff

Mabel Reiff lives on a thirty-acre produce farm in southeastern Pennsylvania with her husband, Ivan, and their children, eight boys and one girl. Green peppers, kale, and red beets keep the bills paid and offer their family lots of (mostly) quality time together during the summer. Her favorite things in life are family, an organized household, books, and cooking for the crowd of growing young men that gathers around their table. On summer mornings she loves those first few moments after five a.m. That's when she takes her cup of coffee and sits on the front porch with her husband to watch the day dawn and talk things over without too many opinions from helpful offspring. The chills of winter winds give her a reason to stay holed up in her house and thoroughly clean and organize everything before she indulges too much in her hobby of writing.

Erica Sauder

Erica Sauder has been told that she is a multi-faceted person, and it might be true. She publishes a small newspaper; enjoys writing, editing, and book-making; does a small bit of photography; occasionally relaxes by piecing quilts; works as a caregiver, cook, and housekeeper at an assisted living home, and tries to find time to clean her tiny house. Some other things she loves: books, lizards, comics, and living in the deserts of New Mexico.

Elfreda Showalter

Elfreda R. Showalter resides in northwestern New Mexico with James, her husband of seventeen years, and ElySandra, her eight-year-old daughter. Elfreda is the sixth child in the King family of seven boys and five girls. A few of Elfreda's favorites are quiet time with God; being at home; heart-to-heart conversations; sunny days with one percent humidity and azure sky; tidy wide-open space; watching birds, butterflies and lizards in the flower garden; plenty of stories and letters to read; and daily writing time. After spending five years in South America and experiencing the pain of no mail for spells of four to six weeks, she rejoices time and again to have a mailbox within sight of her house in the valley between the sandstone cliffs and the river. Life is never boring living with a nature lover daughter and a husband who can speak a couple languages and a phone call away from her many siblings and mother. The Farmington Mennonite Church, where Sasha Krause was kidnapped while she was getting preschool Sunday school books on Saturday evening, January 18, 2020, is seven miles from the Showalter's home. A few weeks after her burial, church services were shut down when COVID-19 swept across the world.

Joel Showalter

Joel Alvin Showalter was born June 6, 1977, in Wingham, Ontario, Canada. In 1992, at the age of fifteen, he moved with his parents to Honduras, Central America, where he continues to reside. He married Marlene

Isabel Gamarra, originally from Agua Azul, Paraguay, on January 6, 1999, and their home has been blessed with five children. Since 1998, Joel has served as a distributor for Mount Zion Literature Ministry, sending Bibles and other Christian literature all over Honduras. He has also worked as a Spanish textbook editor for Rod & Staff Publishers. Currently he is helping to write the Grade 7 Spanish language textbook. Beside these and many other interests and pursuits, he owns a small farm where he grows fine coffee for export to the USA via the JavaTaza company. All are welcome to drop in for a freshly roasted and brewed cup of delicious Honduran coffee!

Crystal Steinhauer

Crystal Steinhauer is from—well, where is she from? Originally from PA, Crystal and family moved to Belize six years ago. Since they returned to the US during the pandemic, they've been sponging off the good graces of their families in Pennsylvania and Ohio, with the intention of returning to Belize when the airport reopens. She and her husband Davy have five children. She blogs about mission life and what she's been learning lately at www.mom-on-a-mission.blog.

Barbie Stoltzfus

Barbie was born in 1977 and lives in Lancaster, PA. She attends the Old Order Amish Church with her scrap dealer husband Elam. Elam and Barbie are blessed with five children ages eight to twenty-one and one son-in- law acquired in the thick of COVID-19. Writing, and crafting make her smile while she tolerates housework. She is a regular writer for *Ladies Journal* and *Shining for Jesus*. She also enjoys writing for Pathway if time allows and is a participant in several writers' workshops. While enjoying every stage of mothering, Barbie openly admits being partial to the middle-aged stage of motherhood. Barbie enjoys mail correspondence and can be reached at 2190 Pequea Lane, Lancaster, PA 17602 or 717-826-7690.

Ruthanna Stoltzfus

Ruthanna Stoltzfus calls a cozy casa in South America home. Life is happiest when she is surrounded by her favorite people- husband Jesse, six precious children and one lovely daughter-in-law. (Her oldest son recently married and lives with his new bride in far-off Pennsylvania.) She and her family moved from PA to Bolivia in 2013. They are busy and fulfilled helping many seeking Russian Mennonite families. She loves coffee and chocolate and hearing from friends.

Dorothy Swartzentruber

Dorothy Swartzentruber lives in southeastern Missouri with her Prince Will and their half-dozen children. A thrift store junkie, she reads voraciously, writes from in the midst of their hillbilly hullaballoo, loves freelance editing, battles to make time to be alone with God, and looks for joy in small things: boyish Lego creations, little-girl songs, bigger-girl bouquets, and rolls of baby fat.

Jane Weaver

Jane Weaver tends towards introversion, has always been a reader and is learning the finer points of being a writer. She enjoys road trips when she doesn't have to drive, bridges and lighthouses for their symbolism, and fabric for its texture. As a wife and mother, she seeks to balance responsibilities with joy.

Sandra Weaver

Sandra Weaver spends her days doing secretary work, helping a teenaged homeschooler, sewing coverings, and writing. She lives at home with her parents and one sister. Her other two siblings live nearby. She enjoys spending time with her two-year-old niece. She loves teaching school, family cookouts, youth volleyball games, curling up by the fireplace with a good book, coffee (day or night), and sitting in a deer stand on a crisp fall day. She may be contacted at coffee.teacherfuel@gmail.com.

Regena Weaver

Regena Weaver lives on six acres in eastern Ontario, where she spends most of her time feeding the family and random neighbors. Sometimes the tables are turned, and friends help put food on her table.

Jessica Yoder

Originally from small-town Colorado, Jessica Yoder now calls the beautiful bustle of Los Angeles home. When she isn't teaching or scheming school, she enjoys meandering her neighborhood streets, reading, and walking with contributors as writing editor at Vibrant Girl magazine. Her writing has appeared in Daughters of Promise and Vibrant Girl. For a glimpse into the world and vision of LA ROAD Christian School, visit laroadchristianschool.com. God is still working there.

Rodney Witmer

Rodney Witmer is a middle-aged husband to Jeanne and the father of six sons. He is the bishop of the Farmington Mennonite Church, a community he has lived in for 35 years. He is a cabinet maker by trade, and owns a small, family-based woodworking business in Aztec, NM.

Judi Zimmerman

Jonas and Judi met in 2018 when Judi went to Farmington, New Mexico to work at The Gingerich Home for the Elderly. Jonas had moved from Missouri in 2013 to help out at Lamp & Light Publishers (also in Farmington), where he is currently employed as printshop manager. Their "I do's" were said on May 29, 2020 in Harrodsburg, Kentucky, where Judi spent twenty two years of her life. Although they would've loved to have all their friends in attendance, neither one of them missed the stress, the crowd, or the vast amount of food prep that COVID-19 graciously allowed them to skip out on, and enjoyed a relaxing outdoor wedding. They have made their home in New Mexico, the beautiful southwest. When they have time to spare, they enjoy reading, grilling, spending time outdoors, or anything they can do to spend time together!

Linda Zimmerman

Linda enjoys life with Bryan, her husband of 23 years, and their two children, Travis-21, and Treva-19. Originally from Lancaster County, PA, they have been on the move. 2003 found them moving to the prairies of Iowa, 2008 to pine trees and cranberry bogs in Wisconsin, 2013 to serve at Faith Mission Home in the VA mountains, and 2018 to rolling cattle country in Northeast Missouri! But they are not stopping there. They have been chosen to move to their church's outreach in 2022, location to be decided. Linda enjoys a good book, baking with sourdough, gardening and canning, times with friends, and a good game of Settlers with her family. She can be reached at 4zgrbj@gmail.com.